Finished Business

Finished Business

Taking care of a loved one with a terminal illness

Donald Gallehr

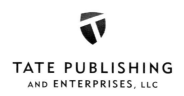

TATE PUBLISHING
AND ENTERPRISES, LLC

Finished Business
Copyright © 2014 by Donald Gallehr. All rights reserved.

No part of this publication may be reproduced, stored in a retrieval system or transmitted in any way by any means, electronic, mechanical, photocopy, recording or otherwise without the prior permission of the author except as provided by USA copyright law.

This book is designed to provide accurate and authoritative information with regard to the subject matter covered. This information is given with the understanding that neither the author nor Tate Publishing, LLC is engaged in rendering legal, professional advice. Since the details of your situation are fact dependent, you should additionally seek the services of a competent professional.

The opinions expressed by the author are not necessarily those of Tate Publishing, LLC.

Published by Tate Publishing & Enterprises, LLC
127 E. Trade Center Terrace | Mustang, Oklahoma 73064 USA
1.888.361.9473 | www.tatepublishing.com

Tate Publishing is committed to excellence in the publishing industry. The company reflects the philosophy established by the founders, based on Psalm 68:11,
"The Lord gave the word and great was the company of those who published it."

Book design copyright © 2014 by Tate Publishing, LLC. All rights reserved.
Cover design by Nikolai Purpura
Interior design by Jomar Ouano

Published in the United States of America
ISBN: 978-1-63418-077-1
1. Health & Fitness / Diseases / Cancer
2. Self-Help / Death, Grief, Bereavement
14.08.04

To those who take care of themselves and others

Contents

Foreword 9

Like Two Kids in a Tree House 13
The Vacation—October 18, 1996 17
The Relationship 21
Childhood 27
South Bridge 33
St. Vincent Hospital 39
Surgery 43
Radiation 51
Chemo 61
First Openings 67
Why? 69
Testing Alternatives 73
A Week in the Hospital 83
Downturn 91
Heartbreak 101

Hospice 109
Hallucinations 117
Meds 127
Blind 137
A Day in the Life Of 143
Physical Therapy 173
Good Times and Getting Out 189
Things Spiritual 197
Death 223
After Death 237

Foreword
by Brendan Gallehr

"Who is Becky Thatcher?" came the volley from the girl's team.

We are back in the early 1990s in my family's living room for a game of Trivial Pursuit. With me on the guys team is my father, brother, and brother-in-law Glen. The girl's team consists of my wife, sister, mother, and my brother's friend Rene.

But the Gallehrs do not play the game like normal people. As part of their mental attack, the girls are already laughing and shouting that the question will go unanswered as they have already flipped the card over to see the answer. The guys start shouting back that not only would the answer equally elude the girls had they been posed the question, but we will find the answer. One person here is not participating in the extra high jinks. My mother sits quietly in her armchair and just watches. I, just like everyone else in the room, know that she had the answer within a second of this Becky Thatcher being mentioned. The girls have a huge advantage as my mother knew the answer to just about every question.

I quickly lean forward and put my elbows on my knees. I try to block out the noise and stare at the floor looking for this mysterious Becky Thatcher. Thatcher, Thatcher, Thatcher. No, not Margaret. But Becky is in my head somewhere.

History…Music…Sports…Literature…Pop Culture…Science…Where is this Becky Thatcher? I continue to quickly flip through the files in my brain. She must be in here somewhere!

As the shouting continues, I slowly look up to see my mother staring at me. The corners of her mouth slightly rise. Yes, she has the answer. I quickly look back down.

If only I could get Margaret Thatcher out of my head. Becky has to be in here somewhere. Perhaps she is Rebecca. But no, the question definitely said Becky. Is she some TV or movie character?

I look back up at my mother. She is still staring at me. I realize that she believes that I should know the answer, and the pressure now lowers on me. She doesn't care about the outcome of the game; she wants me to find this Becky person. The game's outcome is now irreverent to me as the pressure is all on me to not disappoint her on this one single question.

I stare back down. The girls are now shouting that a reasonable time has elapsed. The guys have returned to their drinks and are polling each other on whether to cede defeat on the question.

I ask for just another minute and return to staring at the floor. I can't find Becky.

Thatcher…Thatcher…History…Sports…Music…Becky…Becky…I have to speed up the file flipping in my head. Then the light comes on… "Tom Sawyer's friend," I quietly answer.

The girls sit stunned as the guys start high-fiving. I look over to my mother. And she has the biggest smile on her face. As do I.

As predicted, the girls again end up with another victory that night. Soon, we change the game to everyone against my mother, and she still wins. Now, follow me forward a couple of years. It is a Friday in October and I am off from work. My wife Tracy is quietly studying in our living room. I tell her that I am going to walk down to the mailbox.

Outside it is beautiful. The driveway is about 150 yards long, but I am in no hurry. I look up to see a bright blue sky. Many of the leaves are struggling to keep their green colors, but others have already started to turn into bright yellows, oranges, and reds. There is a slight breeze, but the full sun does mo e than compensate for it.

Reaching the mailbox, I gather the mail and return to my leisurely pace back home. It seems that birds and squirrels are everywhere. A jet is dividing the blue sky above into two with its white trail. Eventually, I reach the side door. I pause to gather in just a little more sun as I walk in.

Tracy is standing in the kitchen with the phone. Holding it forward, she says, "It's your dad. Something is wrong with your mom."

I can hear him talking, but nothing is registering. The blood has left my brain. Tracy helps me to a chair and lowers me into it. She takes the phone back as I then enter the cold and darkness from which I will never return.

Like Two Kids in a Tree House

"What's your favorite song?"
  "Sidewalks of New York."
  "Sidewalks of New York. O.K. What's your favorite movie?"
  "Gone with the Wind."
  "That's interesting. Your favorite actor?"
  "Carry Grant."
  "Actress?"
  "Vivian Leigh."
  "The one who played Scarlet O'Hara?"
  "Yes, and Glenda Jackson."
  "And Glenda Jackson. Elizabeth R. Amazing how she aged. She was almost bald by the end of the movie."
  It is the summer of 1997. Diana and I are home, upstairs in the green bedroom. I am reading questions from *Grandmother Remembers: A Written Heirloom for my Grandchild* given to us by our children. By now Diana is blind from radiation treatments. The doctors had warned us that the radiation had a host of possible side effects, but considering the alternative, that is, allowing the tumor in her brain to return quickly after surgery and kill her, radiation was the right choice. We were bartering for time.
  "Favorite book?"
  "Gone with the Wind."

"Favorite television program?"

"Masterpiece Theater."

I am jotting down her answers on yellow Post-It Notes. I will copy her answers into the book later when I have the time to write clearly. The book is not for me, but for the Grandchildren, two of them now, others to join our family later. Diana is sitting up in a hospital bed we have rented, her hands folded across her lap. Between us is a white dressing table with her medications in a pill divider, and glasses of juice and water. Her black hair flows down to her shoulders, and her cheeks are pink with health, and full. There is no hint of the tumor we know is growing back in the right hemisphere of her brain.

Diana loved watching Masterpiece Theater on Sunday evenings, pieces by Austin, Dickens, and Thackeray, and especially British murder mysteries. She would sit in the living room at the end of the Empire period sofa, her long legs up on the Ottoman, a glass of wine in her hand, piecing together the clues handed out oh so carefully, moving along step by step with the detective to capture the killer.

"Favorite newscaster?"

"Robert MacNeil."

"Of the MacNeil and Lehrer News Hour. Favorite season?"

"Spring."

"Vacation spot?"

"Italy."

I look across the bedroom at the photo on the wall above my mother's block-front desk. Diana and I had vacationed in Italy in 1995, visiting Rome, Florence, Venice, and Milan. In Florence, we climbed a hill to reach one of the Medici residences, then circled behind the massive building to the formal gardens, grand in design and bountiful in roses. Diana sat on a bench to rest, and I took her picture with my portrait lens set on soft focus, her long dark hair flowing across her face in the warm breeze, her skin with a tint of olive coloring, her smile broad, her eyes soft and bright.

In the background rose the hills of Florence with country homes and farms, olive groves and vineyards, family gardens and forests.

I look over at Diana to make sure she is ready to continue. She is remarkably calm in her memories. We both know why I am asking these questions now, but neither of us says.

"Favorite holiday?"

"Christmas."

"Christmas. Not Thanksgiving?"

"No, Christmas. The kids, the presents on Christmas eve, the pizza-roll from Italian Gourmet, the home-made eggnog…"

Diana is quiet. I check to see if she is crying, reach for the tissue box, then pause. There are no tears. Two of our three children had become parents in the last month, events that give Diana enormous pleasure and contentment. She has always loved babies, and when she first held Nicholas, our first grandchild, and then Madeleine, our second, she became quiet as if her every wish had been fulfilled. By then she was already blind, so she saw them only with her fingers, moving them gently across their faces.

I watch until she brings her attention back to the room. "Ready for the next one?"

"Yes."

"Favorite flower?"

"Peonies."

"Peonies?"

Our house was built almost a century ago in 1906 on more than a half acre, with flower gardens and shrubs surrounding the house. Inside the perimeter of the fences are azaleas, hydrangeas, forsythia, weigela, English ivy, periwinkle, acuba, roses, hibiscus, a smoke tree, weeping cherry trees, but only a few scattered peonies. If peonies were her favorite flower, why didn't she plant whole beds of them? We have been married for over thirty-two years, and I am still surprised by her. Even though I am curious, I do not ask. There no point to it for her planting them now is no longer possible, and regret is a luxury we do not need. I am unaware that I am sowing the seeds of another regret—that of not asking her.

"Favorite desert?"

"Ice cream."

"And the last one, what's your favorite saying?"

Together we chant, "If it had teeth, it would bite you," and laugh. Since our first meeting in 1962, Diana has used this expression countless times when I couldn't find something that was right in front of me. Ironically, it also described our marriage. We both spent our lives looking for things that were within easy reach, but we were too blinded by our childhood habits to see them.

As I finish jotting down her last answer, I realize that we are very lucky. Finally, after years of struggle, we are as happy as two kids in a tree house, spending hours together talking, laughing, and taking care of each other.

The Vacation—October 18, 1996

Diana and I took a five-day vacation in Boston over the Columbus Day weekend. On the way, we visited her niece, Amanda, stationed at Otis Field where she served as a medical technician in the Coast Guard. We had always felt close to Amanda, a gentle, beautiful person with a huge heart. We decided to spend a day touring Martha's Vineyard with her, and enjoyed the autumn colors of the island even though it was well past tourist season. On the ferry back to the mainland, Diana fell asleep with the late-afternoon sun on her face. It was very unlike Diana to take naps because they caused her to have trouble sleeping at night. I didn't think much of it, for the rocking of the boat had lulled me into a nap, too.

The next day in Boston, we browsed Mulberry Street antique shops, kitchen stores, and quaint restaurants. We visited my brother, Richard, an engineer who designed machines that plot cardboard boxes, and with him, we toured Harvard, then took pictures of each other standing like tourists; when we walked through Harvard Square, Diana grew tired and sat down on a retaining wall. We were both fifty-four, and in excellent health. We ate well, we exercised, and we did not smoke. I teased her. "Age catching up with you?" Diana smiled. She, too, seemed surprised. We slowed the pace and soon stopped at a pub for a beer. Later that evening, we ate dinner in a cacophonous restaurant, and after the salad, rather than attempt to shout over the din, I reached up with my napkin and blotted a speck of spinach from the left side of her lower lip. After dinner, we said good-bye to my brother and walked back to our bed and breakfast in a beautiful, eighteenth-century row house behind the capitol. Before going to bed, with both hands she raised her left foot and placed it on her right knee before untying her shoelaces. I noticed this unusual gesture but attributed it to her feeling tired. The next morning, Diana said she had dreamed of being in a hospital.

On the morning of October 18, we left Boston to return to our home in Virginia. Within blocks, I was lost. Boston is notorious for decapitated street sign poles, and even residents find themselves making wrong turns. As I glanced down at the map that looked like a plate of blue and green spaghetti, a car behind me honked. I turned down a side street, then pulled over.

I felt confused and embarrassed. "*Damn traffic*," I thought. "*Damn street sign.*" I glanced at Diana who looked as if she were sitting on a beach, watching the waves. How could she not be solicitous, how could she not offer to read the map for me, how could she not search for street signs?

This was a familiar pattern for us. I was feeling inadequate and confused, and yet because these emotions felt so powerful, I didn't know how to express them, and I didn't have enough distance from them to ask her for help.

I glanced again at Diana and thought, "*What are you thinking? Don't you see how lost I am? Don't you see my confusion? Don't you feel my frustration and anger? What the hell are you thinking?*"

I looked back down at the map and thought, "*Why don't you speak?*"

In frustration, I answered my own question by saying to myself, "Oblivious. She's oblivious!"

Eventually, I found my way onto the Massachusetts Turnpike. I was relieved to be out of the city, yet angry at Diana for not helping me when I was in a tough situation. I wasn't about to take responsibility for asking for her help. After all, it was her job to know what I was thinking. Soon we stopped for gas, and Diana bought coffee. It was Diana's turn to drive. Once underway, I read a few papers written by my freshmen, and jotted down comments. When I looked up, I remembered how oblivious Diana had been when I was lost. Even though at the core of me I loved her, I was baffled that she often left me to flounder in difficult situations. It was our pattern. She withheld, I was angry; I was angry, she withheld. I knew I was blaming her, yet I despised her for not helping me. Then I did something I had never done before: I looked at the right side of her head, slightly above her ear, and directed a beam of hatred at it. To this day, I don't know why I did it.

The traffic was light and the day sunny and cool, typical of October in New England. I reclined my seat to rest, closed my eyes, and drifted. I recalled watching *Poltergeist* and felt envious of the couple that sat on the bed and played. We had never done that. When our children were young, they often climbed into our bed, and we played with them, wrestling and tickling, hugging and giggling. Through them we were close to each other, and when they left the nest to go off to college, we were devastated. We had not become strangers as some couples describe their marriages after rearing children; we had never been intimate.

I was between awake and asleep when I felt the car lose power. My first thoughts were, "*The carburetor? Water in the gas?*" I sat bolt upright. The left side of Diana's face was contorted and twitching, and she was reaching her right hand up to stop it. Her eyes were squint shut. She had taken her foot off the pedal, and was steering the car toward the shoulder of the road.

I grabbed the wheel, and slid the shift to neutral. When the car rolled to a stop, I pulled up the brake. For the very first time in thirty-one years of marriage, Diana looked vulnerable. My heart went out to her, and I held her in my arms. "Oh, Sweetie, I love you, I love you. Everything is going to be OK. It's going to be OK."

Her face continued to twitch, and her left leg shook a few minutes more, then stopped. "I'm going to switch seats with you. Can you slide over here?" She nodded. I got out, raced around the car, and helped her to move into the passenger seat. She did not speak. A drop of saliva slid from the left side of her lip. I reached into my pocket and wiped it away with my handkerchief. Then I thought, "*No matter what happens, this is going to change our lives.*"

The Relationship

When you're in love, you see the similarities.

When you're not, you see the differences.

Diana and I both graduated from high school in 1959, Diana from Our Lady of Wisdom Academy Catholic Girls School in Queens, New York, and I from Walden High School in Walden, New York, 75 miles north of New York City. We both took a detour into the religious life—Diana living with the Carmelites in Haiti for four months, and I for one year in the Diocesan Seminary in New York City, then for two years with the Franciscans in Callicoon, New York. Entering the religious life was not uncommon in Catholic families in the 1950's, and like others, we were seeking love. After all, God is love, and what better place to find love than in a religious order?

We left for the same reasons, too. Diana dreamed of men, and of having a family. I dreamed of women. In the end, we both knew we couldn't survive in the religious life.

While I was with the Franciscans, in effect attending the first two years of college, Diana was at Malloy, a Catholic college in New York. Then, in 1962, we both chose St. Bonaventure University for the last two years of college, but for different reasons. Diana was six feet tall, and Bonaventure was not only a basketball school with a huge male-to-female ratio (approximately 2,000 men to

150 women), but some of the men were tall. In addition, she was attracted to the place where Thomas Merton wrote *The Seven Story Mountain*, a charismatic book on the religious aspirations of a young Catholic man who went on to become one of our generation's most famous monks. I chose Bonaventure because it was a Franciscan college; all my credits would transfer, and I liked the Franciscan approach to life.

In September 1962, during orientation of transfer students, we were given a tour of the campus, and it was then that I saw Diana for the first time. She wore a white blouse and blue plaid skirt, typical of someone from a Catholic girls' school. She stood with her arms folded in front of her, her shoulder-length dark-brown hair blowing in the wind, her large, dark-brown eyes looking off into the distance. She looked as beautiful as Jackie Kennedy, only taller and slimmer, with the same square jaw and beautiful complexion. But it was her gaze into the distance that intrigued me the most. What was that woman thinking?

I spent most of my time during my junior year attending classes, writing papers, and studying for exams. I had made close friends in high school and in the seminary, but I didn't seem to click with anyone at Bonaventure. I enjoyed discussions in my literature classes, loved reading Wordsworth, Melville, Shakespeare, and E.E. Cummings, spent hours in the library reading literary critics and writing literary analysis papers in longhand, then pounded them out on my typewriter in my room. I got a part-time job waiting tables in the dining hall, but with little money coming from home, I was poor. Come spring, I had holes in my shoes that I plugged with old index cards from the library. My shirts and slacks were threadbare.

With so few women in our classes, our choices were limited. I dated once in a while on weekends, but only in my senior year did I date anyone regularly, and then half-heartedly, and mostly for companionship. Quite simply, no one interested me.

Then, one night I was planning to attend an off-campus dance with my regular date, but when she caught a cold, she asked Diana to take her place. Diana and I had a good time. I felt mildly awkward dancing with someone who was two inches taller than me, and after several dances, I stood on the first step of the bleacher and said, "I'm as tall as you." While some women might have been offended, Diana took it as playfully as I had intended it, and I liked that. I also liked the banter of our conversation. Years later, while reminiscing about that first date, she said she thought I was nice, sexy, and very masculine.

The next week, I asked her to a movie, and we talked all the way through it. We frequented the Alcove, an Italian restaurant that served my comfort food, spaghetti, with a wonderfully rich marinara sauce. Eventually, we made out, but we did not make love. We were both serious Catholics, and even though I had made love to girls in the past, I held a double standard similar to that of most young men in the fifties and early sixties…we didn't go to bed with girls we thought we might marry.

As couples go, we were boring. We both liked to work, and we often studied together in the library. We were simultaneously serious about school, and playful with each other. We had other similarities: we were Democrats, and coming from working-class backgrounds, held similar views on politics and social issues; we valued education, and considered Bonaventure a good school; we were frugal, I out of necessity, Diana out or temperament, and we never spent more than we had; and, of course, we were both Roman Catholics who had tried the religious life.

Differences other than our height, however, soon emerged, and oddly enough, because we came from families that lacked the ability to talk things out, we were terrible at discussing them. I loved people, loved being in crowds, and liked making friends although I was also shy. Being with people gave me energy. Diana liked small groups or a date with just me, and was happy to be alone. She had friends, even close friends from high school with whom she kept in touch, but she disliked crowds, and when she was surrounded by people, she pulled back like a turtle into its shell.

Even though Diana was a chemistry major, and the brightest student in our graduating class, she also liked history, and took several history classes during her last two years of college. In our last semester, and after we began dating, she took a class on the poetry of Robert Browning, in part to study under Boyd Litzinger, the most renowned professor in the humanities at Bonaventure, and also, I think, to be with me. She treated the class as an afterthought and got her only C in college at a time when such grades were common.

I was an English major, having barely survived required math and science courses. I loved class discussions about the meaning of poems, stories, plays, and novels, and relished talking about ideas. In a good discussion class, I'd sit up front, eager for the give-and-take of opinions. I loved initiating projects, loved starting papers, but wasn't crazy about the details of research. Because Diana was so bright, she breezed through the research, and as the expression goes, she never sweated the details.

A few memories of our college days stand out. One afternoon, we drove up into the mountains to shoot my .22 caliber, Remington target rifle. I had been a National Rifle Association rifle instructor at a children's camp one summer, and I enjoyed shooting at targets. Snow was still on the ground. We hiked a short ways into the woods before setting chips of wood on top of a fallen tree. I showed Diana how to hold the rifle close to her shoulder, how to sight in the target, and how to squeeze the trigger. She laughed with surprise when she took her first shot. She missed, but soon hit the chips, flipping them into the air or downing them behind the log. Quite unexpectedly, and despite the noise of the rifle, a bird sat on the log. Diana swung the rifle and aimed. "Oh no, you don't," I said. She looked at me, devilish and daring. I placed my hand on the rifle and pulled it down. I had seen the same expression of glee in the eyes of my students.

Another memory involves a picnic we went on after dating for about seven months. We took a blanket, a bottle of red wine, a few sandwiches, and several books. Instead of chirping away as we had during our first movie, we were awkward. Diana became very quiet, and I didn't know how to talk to her about her silence. I couldn't figure out what she was thinking, didn't know how to bring up the subject, and couldn't identify my feelings other than to know I felt mighty uncomfortable. Eventually, I became sad, angry, and sullen. I brought it up many years after we were married, and Diana was surprised that I didn't remember the day fondly. If I had to guess, I would say she was being content, and as an introvert, she went inside. I remember it as one of the most awkward days of my life.

Weeks before graduation, my mother died. When I had been home on spring break in March, I noticed that she slept a lot, but I thought she was just tired. She went into the hospital on a Monday and died four days later on Friday. I borrowed my roommate's car and drove home for the funeral. When I returned to Bonaventure, I sat in Diana's car and talked about seeing my mother in a casket, and about not being able to cry for the five days I was home. My emotions had shut down in order to help my family get though the funeral and burial. When I said that, I broke down. Diana put her arms around me, but instead of feeling warm and comforted, I felt cold. Her sympathy was cerebral, and at that moment I physically felt chilly. At the time I was not prone to talk about my emotions, and this arctic chill was enough to shut me down. I did not cry in front of her for years.

The following year, between the end of finals and graduation, I took Diana home to meet my father. Even though they saw each other for only one short evening, they liked each other. The next day, my father went into the hospital. He had been sick with cancer for fifteen years, and sorely missed my mother. That night, when Diana called her parents to tell them that my father had gone into the hospital, they were furious because Diana was would be spending the night in my house alone with me. Her father asked to speak to me, and immediately ordered me out of the house (it was not lost on me that it was my house). Instead of being concerned for my father, he was afraid that his daughter's reputation would be sullied. I was shocked and hurt, but, out of love for Diana, slept in a sleeping bag on the lawn. When I saw her parents several weeks later at graduation, they again berated me for my poor judgment.

The night before graduation, sitting in the front seat of her car, I asked Diana to marry me, mostly because I was afraid of losing contact with her. I was heading to graduate school in New York, and she was taking a job as a researcher at NIH in Washington. She was delighted and said, "Yes." I was terrified. Intuitively, I knew there was something not right between us, but I brushed it aside. In retrospect, I can see that I picked Diana because I loved her, because I thought she would make a great mother to our children, and subconsciously because I thought, with her, I could finish the business of my childhood.

Childhood

From everything I've read about child development, I think we're largely formed by age seven. Early black and white photos show that I was a cute kid, a towhead, and I still have a strand of hair in my baby book. They also show that I was a bit of an extrovert who loved to play the piano and perform in family skits. Those same photos do not show me being held by my mother, and from what I know of her, she did not hold us, hug us, or cuddle with us. Consequently, I grew up hungry for human touch.

My father, a brusque man prone to barking orders, was a third-generation descendent of German immigrants. I have no doubt that he loved us, as I have no doubt that my mother also loved us, but he tended to be dictatorial, or, as we later referred to him, Prussian. I have no recollection of his ever holding a real conversation with me, or of his soliciting my opinion.

My parents had similar backgrounds. Both of them attended the same Catholic school, lived in the same Brooklyn neighborhood, were descendants of German immigrants, and, when the First World War broke out, stopped speaking German in public. After eighth grade, my mother became a secretary, my father became a bookkeeper, and both enjoyed the same social life of the 1920's.

By the early 1930's, my father's hat manufacturing company found it necessary to move out of New York City due to the high cost of labor. It moved about seventy-five miles north of the city to a small town called Walden, (not to be confused with Thoreau's *Walden*, which is outside Boston). Separated from the social life of the city, my father soon became lonely. The story goes that he proposed to my mother by saying, "Would you like to come to Walden to darn my socks." I don't know if the story is true, but knowing my father, chances are it is. He had a small, three-bedroom house built on three-quarters of an acre on the edge of town, half a mile from work, and turned the backyard into a huge vegetable garden, no small feat for a city boy. I came along in 1941 after my older brother and sister, and was followed by my younger sister. The family prospered throughout the forties until my father was diagnosed with throat cancer in 1950. He was one of the early radiation patients, and although his cancer was burned into extinction, the left side of his neck looked like tenderloin. He lived for another fifteen years, but his health was never good. He lost part of his hearing, and had frequent bouts of painful ear infections. At the same time, my mother suffered from a lack of energy that everyone thought was a result of having four children and several miscarriages. She died in 1964, a year before my father. In 1996, we learned that she had hemochromatosis, a disease that produces excessive blood and makes a person lethargic.

My father was a happy man, and enjoyed having children. Unfortunately for us, he ordered rather than asked. My brother made him a wooden sign that read, "The Boss," and my father displayed it with pride on top of the television. We ate most dinners in silence listening to Drew Pearson and the News on the radio, and only a few meals do I recall his being warm-hearted and conversational. My mother, in addition to having hemochromatosis, was not, as they say, a warm fuzzy. I once brought home a girlfriend who placed her hand on my mother's arm, a simple gesture of friendship. My mother recoiled. Not only do the photos in the family album not show her holding us, I have no recollection of her giving us hugs. I came home from school one day and was mystified that my dog, a great dane we had named Ajax, was not around to greet me. I went calling and searching for him, and eventually found his body across the street, his intestines lying beside him. I ran back to the house and into the kitchen where my mother was standing behind an ironing board, ironing clothes. "Can't we put his stomach back in?" I asked her. She did not move out from behind the ironing board, she did not say she was sorry, and she did not hug me. Instead, she surmised that he had been hit by a car, and continued to iron.

Diana's parents also came from New York. Her grandfather, Willie Batch, ran off to play professional baseball while his son, Ed, Diana's father, was still young. Her grandmother, May, raised him with the help of her parents. Diana's father was convinced that his father would return on his twenty-first birthday, so he dressed up and waited. His father never showed up. Like my father and mother, Diana's father had an eighth grade education, and even though he showed talent as an artist, his mother decided against sending him to art school. He took a job in the printing business and learned to fly a plane. He knew Lindberg and Earhart, but gave up flying when he got married. He was one of the most handsome men I have ever met, and from him, Diana got her good looks and intelligence.

Diana's mother's family was Irish, had many children, and owned a dairy farm in up-state New York. When her grandfather died, her grandmother brought the family to the city and became a policewoman, a sizable accomplishment at the time. Diana's mother had various jobs before meeting her father, then settled down to raise Diana and her two younger brothers. They moved around New York and Long Island, selling their houses when someone gave them a good offer. In the early 1960's, they moved to Virginia for the same reason my father's company had moved out of New York, to avoid the high cost of labor.

I remember her parents going to see the movie *Tom Jones* and walking out because of the sex scenes. Her father was surprised that we considered our walking out as prudish. I also remember Diana telling stories of her father being quite angry with her brothers, pushing the kitchen table at them to pin them to the wall while she trembled behind the door. Even though he never reprimanded her, she did come away from her childhood with an inordinate fear of her father's anger.

The night before Diana and I were married, I couldn't sleep. I stood at the window of the hotel starring out at the parking lot like a glossy-eyed, night watchman. I was making a decision I couldn't reverse because divorce was not an option for my Roman Catholic mind. I felt trapped. I had done everything right. I had dated and courted Diana, I had refrained from having intercourse, I had asked her to marry me, I had asked her father for her hand, I had participated fully in every part of the wedding plans. Yet, I felt like I was driving through a fog that wouldn't lift, a fog that was coming from somewhere inside me. Something was wrong, but I couldn't put my finger on it.

After the wedding and reception, we went back to Diana's parents' house for pictures, then changed into our honeymoon clothes, and drove out of Winchester, Virginia, toward Washington, D.C., where we were to spend our wedding night. Diana became silent, almost withdrawn, as if someone had dimmed the light switch. I was nervous about this huge step we had taken, and tried to make small talk. It was as if I were playing catch with her, but she wasn't returning the ball. I was baffled. This was to be our happiest day, and yet we were clearly not happy.

That evening, we ate dinner at the restaurant in the hotel. I ate the entree, wiped my lips with the napkin, folded it and placed it on the table. Diana ate the appetizer, the salad, the entree, and the dessert. Eventually, we walked almost single file from the restaurant to the room. I used the bathroom first, then waited as I heard her wash her face, brush her teeth, brush her hair, and slip into her nightgown. When she came out, she was beautiful.

We made love with awkward gentleness, then lay side by side, staring at the ceiling. Before sliding into sleep, I said, "Your mom said it might take six months before we're comfortable with each other." Diana was quiet, but patted my hand. In silence, I prayed it would take no longer. It never occurred to me that she might be afraid of sex.

Over the years, Diana and I meshed in some very important ways. We held the same values on family, child rearing, education, politics, money, and religion. The strength of our marriage came from these similarities.

We clashed in some very important ways, too. If you put the two of us together in a room, we didn't know what to do. We were awkward with each other when left alone.

As with most couples, we lugged the unfinished baggage of our childhood into our marriage. Because my mother did not hold or hug me, I craved being touched, and yet at the same time being touched was strange and threatening to me. The scene of my mother standing behind the ironing board became a powerful image for me of the emotional deprivation of my childhood.

Diana's unfinished business was opening her heart. Somewhere in her childhood, her heart closed, and even though she loved our children and me deeply, she loved more with her head than her heart. I think it is quite possible that her controlling image became the scene with her father shouting at her brothers.

When we clashed, Diana would do whatever she could to get me angry, to once again experience that horrible scene from her childhood. And I would do whatever I could to engineer an emotionless response. We had become our own worst enemies. Several times in the 1980's and 1990's we tried to work things out through marriage counseling, but in fact nothing worked.

South Bridge

I drove off the Massachusetts Turnpike and stopped at a diner for directions to the nearest hospital. "It's the next exit up the turnpike," a waitress said, pointing up the road. As I turned around to leave, the waitress followed me to the door and gawked at Diana reclining in the passenger seat. I hated that. Yes, we were having an emergency, but I didn't like the waitress starring at Diana as us as if we were in a movie. It was then I noticed I had left the car in drive with the brake on. I was more nervous than I thought.

    I swung back on the turnpike and sped toward Boston to the South Bridge exit, where a small hospital lay a few miles into the town. It felt strange to drive straight up to the emergency entrance. "This is an emergency," I told myself. "You have a right to drive up here." I held Diana's left arm, much like a policeman holds the arm of someone he has arrested, and we walked to the receptionist's window. She quietly jotted down our insurance information, and as we both answered the questions, I noticed that Diana seemed remarkably calm. I may have looked calm on the outside, but inside I was terrified. We then walked back to the emergency room to enter a cubicle, and Diana then laid on the bed.

Diana's father had had a stroke in the early 1970's, and he was left partially paralyzed on his left side. I remembered his sitting in the front hallway of his large, antebellum rented house in Winchester, in a wheel chair, in the sun, philosophic and glad to be alive. I was hoping Diana's situation would be no more serious than that.

When the nurse entered, I blurted out, "I think it might be a stroke." I desperately wanted to know what was wrong. The nurse ignored my comment and took Diana's pulse, blood pressure, and temperature. No doubt she had seen her share of husbands like me. Her silence told me I didn't know what I was talking about. The nurse left, and Diana and I were alone.

A short-harried woman bustled into the cubicle. "Hello, I'm Dr. Morris. What do we have here?" I told her what happened in the car, and added, "Do you think it might be a stroke?"

"No, but it might be Bell's Palsy. Was she driving with the window open, with the air rushing against her face? Sometimes a sustained cool breeze will temporarily paralyze the facial nerve that runs beneath the ear down to the muscles of the face."

Why was she talking to me? Diana was right there. Why didn't she ask Diana?

"The window was open for only a few minutes. She doesn't like breezes blowing on her face." Now I was playing this weird game. Before I could finish, Dr. Morris was called out to attend to another patient. How could someone else be more important, more in danger, more in need of help? I looked down at Diana. She was breathing, but she was not bleeding; she just looked stunned. Dr. Morris's quick departure forced me to step back, to look beyond our small cubicle.

Diana lay still, looking off into the distance. Perhaps she, too, was thinking about others. I felt awkward with her silence, and I, myself, didn't know what to say.

Dr. Morris returned after what seemed a great while. "The MRI mobile unit is here, and the first appointment is open. I think it would be good to check things out." It didn't take much to add things up. She didn't know what was the matter with Diana. I didn't know, Diana didn't know, so we were looking for a machine to give us an answer.

The nurse returned to lead the way, then turned to Diana and said, "Why don't we use the wheel chair, just in case?"

Just in case? In case she might have another whatever it was? I wheeled Diana down the corridor to the MRI unit, and it felt like I was wheeling her to the electric chair.

When we reached the mobile unit reception area, a technician said, "She'll need to remove her wedding ring, necklace, and earrings to prevent interference with the magnets." *What is this?* I could feel a shift in our identity, much like feeling the tremors of an impending earthquake. We were no longer on stable ground. For over thirty years, we had defined ourselves with what these objects represented. How many times had we placed an *X* in the box "Married." And while the jewelry was by no means priceless, it did say we were not poor. I had bought her small diamond engagement ring while still in graduate school at a time when I was truly poor. Years later, due in large measure to Diana's salary which exceeded my own, I was able to buy her a nice sterling silver necklace from Tiffany's, and then a year later matching earrings. As Diana removed her jewelry, I felt like I was slipping back in time, before our years of prosperity.

Within minutes, the technician reappeared. "We're ready," she said.

I turned to Diana, and said, "I love you."

"I love you, too." She stood and walked the few steps into the trailer. The door shut behind her.

I looked around. I was standing in a waiting room where magazines were piled in stacks on short tables beside chairs. *Do people actually read magazines in situations like this!* I sat in a chair, stood up, sat down, stood up. The magazines had cover stories about losing weight, celebrities breaking up, how to improve your sex life, recipes for the perfect Thanksgiving. They all seemed so frivolous. I wanted to talk to a technician who whisked through the waiting room. I wanted answers. I wanted this suspense to go away, just go away.

Fifteen minutes later, Diana returned, ashen. She sat in the wheel chair, silent as stone. I rolled her back to the emergency room to wait for the results, and there exchanged filler sentences about Boston, the kids, and our jobs. Finally, a nurse brought a large brown envelope to Dr. Morris who was standing at the nurse's station. Dr. Morris opened the envelope, slid out the MRI, took one look at it. Then, in a gesture I will never forget, she slapped it against her thigh.

"That's not good," Diana said. Dr. Morris rushed over to us with consternation and disgust, and with a strange tone of apology in her voice, asked us to fellow her into a small waiting room. Dr. Morris began to cry.

"What is this?" I thought. *"You're the doctor. Doctors aren't supposed to cry. Patients cry."*

Amid tears, she looked at Diana and blurted out, "You have a tumor!" She held up the MRI.

The MRI looked like an x-ray. I could see the tumor, a baseball-sized, white mass, smack in the middle of her right hemisphere, pushing the corpus callosum of her brain into her left hemisphere, much like the indentation of a guard rail after an accident. I had studied the structure of the brain in connection with left-brain, right-brain thinking, so I knew the corpus callosum was supposed to divide the hemispheres in a straight line. Something was really wrong here. I didn't know if the tumor was considered large or small, I didn't know if it were life threatening, and I didn't understand why Dr. Morris was so upset. I had never seen a doctor cry. I thought she might have been distraught from a sleepless night in the emergency room.

"Is it benign?" I asked.

"I don't know," she said, "I can't tell from the MRI. It has to be removed. It doesn't matter if it's malignant or benign."

"I'm sorry," she added, then left. We were numb.

This is it, I thought. *Not just a moment in time, but a life-defining moment.* I looked down at Diana, stunned into silence. I felt so sorry for her, so drawn to her helplessness. "I love you," I told her. I held her in my arms, then blurted out, "All I ever wanted to do was fall in love with you." It would be months before I realized the second meaning of this statement: that after thirty-two years of marriage, even though I loved her, I had still not fallen in love with her.

"I love you, too," she said.

There was one phone in the room but a woman, distraught and weeping, was using it. I rolled Diana back into the hall to use a pay phone. I called our son John, a doctor at the University of Kentucky med school in his fifth year of residency. He was not in Lexington, so the nurse gave me his number at a clinic in rural Kentucky where he worked on Fridays. I called the clinic and left a message. "Please have John return our call. This is an emergency." I had always been very careful about not using the word "emergency" to get in touch with our children, so by using it now he would know it clearly was urgent.

He called back within minutes, and I told him what I knew. I also told him that Dr. Morris had recommended our going to St. Vincent Hospital in Worcester, a teaching hospital, about thirty miles away, in case Diana needed surgery. "Can you fly to Boston?" I asked him. "My brother should be able to meet you at Logan airport and drive you to St. Vincent."

"Yes," he said, strong and confident. I was greatly relieved. We were very close to our children, and the thought of having John with us was very comforting.

We then called our son, Brendan, a manager of a car dealership in Fairfax, Virginia. Friday was his day off, and he had just walked down his driveway to collect the mail. Our daughter-in-law, Tracy, answered the phone, then turned it over to Brendan. Immediately, he offered to come to Massachusetts. "No, we don't know what we're doing yet," I told him. I put Diana on, and she said, "I'm OK. Don't worry, honey."

We called our daughter, Marisa, an attorney with a law firm in Washington, D.C. She said, "Oh my God! Is she going to die?"

"I don't think so," I said, "at least not from this tumor." I had no way of knowing what would happen, but I didn't want to admit that the tumor might be serious. I handed the phone to Diana.

"I'm fine. Don't worry about me." It was typical Diana, solicitous of other people, even when she was having a difficult time. I felt relieved that we weren't in this alone.

We rolled back into the cubicle where the nurse started an IV. "What's that for?" I asked.

"Dilantin. It controls seizures. And this one is Decadron. It will shrink the tumor. Less likely to have seizures." I finally made the connection. Diana suffered a seizure, not a stroke.

Dr. Morris came in. "I think it best that Diana go to St. Vincent in an ambulance so that she has medical help if anything happens." It wasn't a real choice. Of course I didn't want anything to happen. One seizure on the turnpike was enough. Within minutes, two burly emergency medical technicians shifted Diana from the cubicle bed to the ambulance gurney.

"You're a tall drink of water," one said. At six feet and 145 pounds, she stretched the length of the gurney. After a short wait, they rolled her into the ambulance. When the closed the doors, I ran over to our Camry and followed. The drive in the heavy, late Friday afternoon, traffic at thirty-five miles per hour seemed to take forever. A few hours ago, she was sitting in the car, and now she was flat on her back in an ambulance. I was aware of being very tense.

"No need to speed," I said aloud to myself. "The emergency is over." It was as if I exhaled for the first time in hours.

St. Vincent Hospital

I followed the ambulance up to the emergency entrance of St. Vincent Hospital, parked the car, and ran around as they unloaded Diana, with caring, with expertise, but nevertheless, like a slab of meat. During the hour we spent in the corridor waiting for our room, I talked with the medical technicians, swapping stories I had heard from John when he was a teenager working for the rescue squad. Diana, laying on the gurney, was subdued. The drugs were making her sleepy, and, as I learned much later, seizures leave people confused and disoriented.

We spent the evening on the phone calling friends and relatives. The doctors and nurses were solicitous and caring, offering to help in this new world that was so foreign to us.

John arrived after midnight, driven from the airport by my brother, Richard. I hugged him like a close friend I hadn't seen in years, feeling as if I now had a powerful and compassionate ally against this thing that had exploded our lives, someone who could answer our countless questions and talk to us at length. In some ways this was not new. We had enormous admiration for our children, and always found great comfort in their company.

John came to the room and talked briefly to Diana. I had a vague sense that he was talking to her not only as a son, and also as a doctor, listening for signs that only doctors read. "I have to leave you for a few minutes to take a look at the MRI," I told Diana. "We'll be right back. Are you going to be OK without us?"

"Yes, I'm fine," she said. I hated leaving her alone.

Richard, John, and I walked down the hall to the nurses' station. For the first time since the seizure, I felt so comforted. John was 6'2" with long arms and legs from Diana's side of the family; his sandy, blonde hair and fair skin came from mine. He was handsome; good looks came from both sides.

Once at the nurse's station, John slid the MRI up under the clip of the light box, and in a way I had not known before, I saw him as a doctor. It was a simple action, but for me, significant and reassuring. I learned much, much later, only when writing this, that when John looked at the MRI, he thought the tumor looked bad. At the time he said nothing, not wanting to alarm us.

When we returned to the Diana's room, I leaned over the hospital bed railing and said, "Everything is going to be OK. The tumor has to come out, but we have options about where to have the operation. We could stay here in St. Vincent and have the tumor removed in the next day or two; we could go to Mass. General in Boston, which has some of the best surgeons in the country; or we can return to Virginia—to Charlottesville or Fairfax. We'll be talking to Dr. Stone, the neurosurgeon here, in the morning to see what he thinks. Is that OK?" I imagined Diana already felt helpless, so I wanted to keep her informed, to include her in decisions.

"Yes, it's OL," she said, and patted my hand.

That short night Diana slept in the hospital bed, while John, Richard, and I slept on the floor.

At 6:30 the next morning, Dr. Bernard Stone, John, and I reviewed the MRI and discussed our options. Dr. Stone was a Santa Clause of a doctor, with a balding head, white hair, and a gentle handshake. I felt comfortable with him as a person and surgeon, and if we had chosen him to do the surgery at St. Vincent, I would have felt safe. As we talked, it became clear that the tumor did not have to come out immediately. Diana's seizure was under control, and her heart and breathing were not being affected by the tumor. I learned later that it is rare for a tumor to grow so fast that it would have to be removed when first discovered.

After talking to Diana, we decided to return to Virginia because the doctors there were excellent, and we would be closer to home. Having family nearby was very important to us. We chose Fairfax over Charlottesville because it was only 35 miles from home, three miles from Marisa's apartment, and two miles from Diana's work. We did not know until later that it was among the top 20 hospitals in the country for oncology. At the time, I did not know that oncology was the study of cancer.

We left St. Vincent Hospital around 9:00 AM. John wanted to drive, so I sat in the back, and Diana sat in the passenger seat. Even though we had Dilantin and Decadron pills with us to control the seizures, I was scared. While driving through Connecticut, John turned to Diana and said, "Ma, this time it really is all in your head." The three of us laughed.

We stopped at a gas station in New Jersey for lunch, and to give John a chance to call Fairfax Hospital. He talked to an admissions nurse who recommended a surgeon who best fit Diana's needs. John then called the surgeon who arranged for Diana to be admitted. I did not know at the time, but if John had not made these arrangements, Diana would have entered through the emergency room, a procedure that would have taken hours. We arrived at Fairfax at 5:30 p.m., and because of John's calls, Diana was in a room within fifteen minutes. It felt so, so good to be back in Virginia.

Later that evening, Marisa and her husband Glen, and Brendan and his wife Tracy, came into Diana's room at Fairfax Hospital with balloons, flowers, and cards. It was the closest I came to crying since Diana's seizure. There is something wonderful about the love of one's family, something that surpasses everything else.

Surgery

When John called ahead to Fairfax Hospital to prepare for admission, he had asked for the names of brain surgeons, and the hospital referred him to Doctors Azzam and Dennis. Both partners would look at the MRI on Monday.

By now we knew that most brain tumors have to be removed because the brain is affected by even the slightest invasion. If you're lucky and the tumor is benign or harmless, it needs to be removed only if it is growing or impeding neurological or bodily functions. We were hoping to be lucky, but we already knew her tumor had caused not only the seizure on our way back from Boston, but also tiredness (within the last year, she fell asleep from exhaustion around 9:00 p.m. almost every night), and numbness in her lower left lip. That is why she couldn't feel the speck of salad I removed when we were in Boston.

John told us that there were four types of brain cancer, with type one being the most benign, and type four the most malignant. Types three and four were considered life threatening. He said that some tumors grow so slowly that they did not threaten the life of the patient. Once removed, they are either gone forever, or if part of them remains, they grow back so slowly that another surgery years down the road keep them in check. We had no idea when Diana's tumor started, and we had no way of knowing whether it was a type that grew fast or slow, or even if it were malignant or benign without first removing a piece of it for a pathologist to look at under a microscope.

In the morning, Dr. Azzam came to the room and introduced himself to us, and almost immediately he asked to see the MRI from Southbridge hospital. He held it up to the window and said, "It looks like a type three or four." I felt numb. Something was wrong. I could hear his words, but I couldn't believe them. I looked over at Diana sitting on the bed, crying quietly. I held her hand and rubbed her arm. I looked up at the white ball on the MRI, and wanted Dr. Azzam to be wrong, wanted the tumor to be type one, wanted someone to take it out, take it all out, and go away so we could resume our lives.

After he left, Diana said, "That's not good news."

"No," I said. "But he may be wrong. We'll be getting a second opinion from Dr. Dennis. His might be better." I patted her hand, reassuring myself as much as her. I can't say it was wisdom that prompted me to fill the void of ignorance with optimism. I just couldn't face the possibility that this tumor might prove fatal.

Dr. Dennis visited later in the day. He had a square jaw and black hair, and reminded me of the Irish priests of my childhood. I could see Diana's Irish ancestry in the clean lines of his face, and liked him immediately. His handshake was strong and firm.

He held the MRI up to the window as Dr. Azzam had, and, with the confidence of one reading the front page of *The New York Times*, said, "It's a type one or two." I smiled, and liked him even more. Diana was smiling, too. But how could this be? Dr. Azzam and Dr. Dennis were partners. They were reading the same MRI. They were in the hard sciences, not the arts where things are open to interpretation.

"Are you guys playing good cop, bad cop?" I asked.

I expected him to laugh. He didn't. Instead, he took out his Montblanc pen and pointed to the area around the tumor, the very area Dr. Azzam had pointed to. "It's definitely type one or two, but we have to wait for surgery to be certain." Ah, both partners were guessing. It would be up to the pathologist and his microscope to decide. Dr. Dennis cleared his throat. "If it's type one, the surgery could be curative." My smile broadened. Curative, as in a cure, as in it would go away, go completely away, and leave us alone.

"Which of you will do the surgery?" I asked.

"I will," he said. I liked this man. I knew it made no sense to think that if Dr. Dennis performed the surgery, the tumor would be benign, yet how could I avoid the connection. I wanted the good guy to win. At the very least, his optimism would give us several days of hope, a commodity in scarce supply of late.

"We've scheduled the surgery for 8:00 Thursday morning. I see no reason for you to stay here."

"We can go home?" I was elated. I turned to Diana. What? She looked frightened. What is she thinking? This is good news. Why isn't she happy? We could go home for three days. Home is where we're safe.

I looked back at Dr. Dennis. He, too, was looking at Diana. "The medications will control the swelling in the brain and prevent seizures." He had read her face and was reassuring her even though she hadn't said a word.

"Thank you," I said. I shook his hand, his strong hand, the very hand that would search for, find, and destroy the tumor. Search and destroy, like soldiers in war.

The next morning we packed up and left. I felt like a caged hawk being set free.

Tuesday evening, at home, Diana seemed more relaxed, and I noticed color returning to her olive complexion. Our neighbor, Rocky, who trained and rode her own horses in steeplechase races, brought flowers, Marisa cooked dinner, and Diana mended John's sweater. I walked about like a soldier in no-man's land caught between the lines. Would the next shot come from the right, from the left, from behind? That night, Diana slept for 10 hours, and I had to wake her to give her her medications.

On Wednesday, Diana, John, and I walked through the park in balmy, 65-degree weather. Our pace was slow and careful. No one would guess that Diana had a grenade-sized tumor in her head. We ate lunch at a local Chinese restaurant, and at Diana's request, Marisa cooked flank steak for dinner. Was this comfort food? Her family had flank steak on special occasions, usually when entertaining. Or was she preparing her system for surgery. Diana looked scared and didn't talk much about her feelings. She told John while sitting on the porch and basking in the sun that she felt nervous and confused. Perhaps this was the seizure talking. By now, I attributed her silence after her initial seizure to disorientation. She knew where she was, what day it was, but was less certain of other things. I began to think of seizures in electrical terms, short circuiting the usual pathways in the brain. Because Diana did her thinking on the inside, we did not get to see the extent of her confusion, other than more prolonged silences.

When I began keeping a journal in 1979, I also introduced our three children to this practice, in part as self-defense (they would have no desire to peek at mine if they, too, were keeping one), and in part I hoped that they find self-discovery as enjoyable as I did. To entice them, I offered them a quarter per day for writing a minimum of one page. Of the three, only John continued to keep a journal. Wednesday night, he later told me, he wrote, "The numbness in her lower lip is resolved." Several months before her seizure, he, too, had noticed that she had left a bit of salad sticking to her lower left lip. The drug Decadron was now shrinking her tumor, thus releasing its pressure on her brain, and allowing sensation to return.

On Thursday, John, Diana, and I left the house at 6:00 a.m. and drove to Fairfax Hospital. We entered the large waiting room with its attractive artwork and comfortable sofas. The hospital allowed only one person to be with the patient during pre-op, so John waited upstairs while Diana and I rode the elevator two floors down. I would return to the waiting room to be with John during surgery.

As Diana changed into a hospital gown, I noticed her back. As kids, we described belly buttons and spines as "innies" or "outies." Diana's spine was an outie. The gown itself must have been designed for the convenience of the surgeon because it left little dignity for the patient. Diana laid on the gurney and looked at the ceiling. Small talk had always been difficult for us. I held her hand, cold as marble from fear, and we talked about the Monet painting on the wall. Then we were silent. We talked about Fairfax Hospital having an excellent reputation for treating cancer. Then we were silent. We said we were not afraid of the surgery. Then we were silent. We were worried, and stopped talking altogether.

A thin, young man slid the curtain aside. "I'm Dr. Peterson, your anesthesiologist." He leaned over and examined Diana's arms. "You have great veins." John's med-school friend, Dan Ness, also an anesthesiologist, had made the same remark at dinner the night before John graduated from med school. It was true—her veins were prominent, and easy to find. I smiled. Even though her veins had nothing to do with the outcome of the surgery, I wanted the surgery to proceed smoothly. And, I was starving for something positive. Dr. Peterson pierced the vein on her left arm, and adjusted the drip from the plastic bag on the pole. When Dr. Peterson was finished, he left, and we again gazed at the Monet. "Does it hurt?" I asked.

"No, it's OK."

A nurse came in. "It's time," she said, and unlocked the wheels of the gurney to roll Diana into the operating room.

I leaned down and kissed Diana. "I love you," I said.

"I love you, too."

I sat down next to John in the waiting room. He said it would be a routine operation with microscope, microsurgical instruments, and microsurgical procedures, much like the surgeries broadcast on television. He said the technical name for any operation involving opening the skull is craniotomy. "Dr. Dennis will make an incision into the scalp, and then will remove a piece of bone to gain access to the tumor. Once he removes the tumor, he will replace the bone and sew the scalp back together." John's calm words and soft tone reassured me. "The reason for surgery is that it is the most effective treatment for brain tumors, especially for tumors that are in parts of the brain that can be cut or removed without damage to the brain. It is also the least invasive."

"How so?"

"Radiation and chemotherapy are less precise. Dr. Dennis will try to remove the whole tumor because, depending on the type, any remaining parts will grow back. If it is a type, one tumor, and if Dr. Dennis is successful in getting it all out, that will be the end of it." That was exactly what I was hoping would happen.

John O'Connor, a long-time close friend and colleague, stopped by. He said he felt unsettled because Diana was the first of our generation to have a potentially serious illness. "I'm sorry I haven't kept in touch with you guys," he said. Like me, his teaching and administrative duties kept him very busy, and neither of us had stayed in touch with the many friends we had developed earlier in our careers. It was good to see him.

Around 11:30, John O'Connor left and Marisa joined us. Soon after, Dr. Dennis walked in, with his dark hair wet and his skin ruddy, looking like a rugby player after a scrum. "The surgery went well, but the tumor is not a type one as I hoped. It is either a type two or three, and possibly type four. The lab will be able to tell which." Type two or three. Not as good as type one, but still not as bad as type four. The radiation and chemotherapy will kill the rest of the tumor. Not the best news, but not the worst. We can get this thing yet.

I looked over at John and saw tears in his eyes. Why is he crying. Surely, this can be fixed. Dr. Dennis' news isn't that bad. John's reaction doesn't make sense. What is wrong here?

Dr. Dennis left, Brendan arrived a few minutes later, and immediately we were paged. Diana was in the recovery room.

John, Brendan, Marisa, and I descended the elevator, and walked past the large, central nurse's station to see her sitting up on a gurney, her head wrapped in a bandage and she had an IV in her arm. She introduced her nurses to us by name. Considering she had just undergone brain surgery, I was amazed and relieved by the accuracy and gracefulness of her introductions. Brendan whispered to me, "She always remembers people's names." As far as I could tell, she had come out of surgery without any damage.

"How was the operation," she asked.

"It went well," we said. "She didn't ask about the type of tumor, and we didn't tell her."

"We knew it was bad and she didn't," John later told me he had written in his journal. She then described to us in detail the Monet in pre-op. It was typical Diana—in the midst of chaos or tragedy, a calm reference to something beautiful.

The nurse motioned to us that it was time for us to go, time to let her rest. The hospital was unusually crowded, so Diana spent the day in post-op. John, Brendan, Marisa, and I spent the afternoon at Marisa's apartment only a few miles from the hospital, and John and Marisa downloaded material for us to read about brain cancer from the *Mayo Clinic Family Health* book. We visited Diana later in the afternoon, and that night I slept at Marisa's. It was the last night I would sleep apart from Diana. I was scared.

Radiation

Friday morning, the day after surgery, Diana was moved from the recovery room upstairs to a room on the "floors" as the nurses referred to them. I arrived at 10:00 in the morning and was so glad to see her. As irrational as it was, I thought she would be safe if I could be with her. In reality, it was I who was feeling safe by being with her. For the remainder of the morning, we did the usual hospital things while awaiting a visit from the oncologist.

From talking with John and reading the *Mayo Clinic Family Health Book*, I had learned about brain cells, nerve cells, and cancer cells. To steel myself against the worst news, I studied grade four tumors that grow in a type of brain cell called a glial, and more specifically a glial cell called an astrocyte because it is shaped like a star. When an astrocyte becomes cancerous, that is, when it grows out of control like kudzu, it is called an astrocytoma. Astrocytomas are the most common of brain tumors, and grade four astrocytomas are considered deadly because they cannot be totally removed with surgery, and because they spread so quickly into neighboring tissues. Dr. Dennis said Diana's tumor wasn't a grade one, and probably wasn't even a grade two, so I was hoping for grade three, and dreading a grade four.

The nurses told us that Dr. Binder would be our oncologist, and that he would bring with him the results of the lab tests. He arrived after lunch. He was a handsome man, with slightly grey hair, a smartly tailored suit, and a New England dialect. We shook hands, and with the directness of a New Englander, he said, "Your tumor is glioblastoma multiforme, a type four astrocytoma." I felt as if I had been punched. I wanted air. I wanted control. I couldn't move my head to look at Diana.

"What's the prognosis?" I asked, caught up in his directness.

"One to three years," he said. Another punch. The air was gone.

Dr. Binder described the benefits of radiation and chemotherapy as if he were delivering a sales pitch. At the time, I resented it. Is that how he could afford expensive suits? What a shitty job he had, selling chemo to people who were going to die anyway. I struggled to listen to him, pushing away my resentment. Without radiation and chemotherapy to retard the inevitable return of the tumor, Diana would live, at most, only another five months. We needed something.

"Does alternative medicine have anything that can deal with this?" I asked.

"No," he said.

I was shocked by the bluntness of his answer. I wanted to punch back. I wanted to get rid of him and the tumor at the same time. I had grown up in the North where bluntness is common, but after 30 years of living in the South, I was accustomed to the Southern prelude, the acknowledgment of the other person and the situation, for after the prelude, and only after the prelude, was the truth delivered. I wanted him to console us, to tell us that all this would go away, to say he understood. I wanted him to soothe the pain, to soften the news. Later, much later, I came to appreciate his honesty. There was no sense in telling anything but the truth, and no matter how you sliced it, the truth was all there was.

I finally turned my head and looked at Diana. She was sitting on the bed, her head bandaged from surgery, asking questions and listening to answers. She looked composed, as if she were deciding to transplant the peonies. When I returned my attention to Dr. Binder, I heard him talking about the importance of the quality of Diana's life, that it was not worth turning her into a vegetable to survive an additional unknown number of months. I had known for years that people talk about the quality of life only when there is no hope of recovery. I understood, in a way I had not known when he delivered the prognosis that he knew she would die.

Before he left, he said Dr. Susan Pierce, a radiation oncologist, would visit us. "She is a wonderful doctor, one who other doctors admire and respect." I shook hands with him, Diana shook hands with him, and we said good-bye. I turned back to Diana.

"You turned white," she said.

"No wonder," I said. "Where's John?" John had stood beside me throughout our discussion with Dr. Binder, asking questions quietly.

"He left. I think he went down the hall to the waiting room to tell the others." Diana was handling the news better than I.

When Dr. Pierce arrived, she folded her hands behind her back and leaned against the wall. Her voice was soft and gentle, yet also scientific and factual. I wanted her take care of us. Instead, she spoke about the quality of life, about the duration of the radiation treatments, and about the possible side effects. Diana's hair might fall out, her scalp might dry and turn red around the treated areas, fluid might buildup in her ears, and she might go deaf. The radiation might burn healthy brain tissue, and she might lose her memory. She might throw up. Her blood pressure might drop. She might get dizzy. Her face may flush, and she may lose control of her kidneys. She might have problems breathing, and a lung might collapse, and she'll probably lose weight, and get depressed. She might even die from radiation. Dr. Pierce held nothing back.

I knew a little about radiation from my father's throat cancer. He had smoked over two packs of cigarettes a day for years, and the cobalt treatments were stronger than needed, burning not only the cancer, but also healthy tissue in the left side of his neck. He lived another 15 years, and in addition to his having suffered very painful earaches, he was forced to purge the acrid-smelling rotten tissue each morning and evening with a saltwater solution that he forced through his nose. Radiation had saved my father from death, but left him sick. To say the least, I had very mixed views of this therapy.

Dr. Pierce said we had the option of taking part in a research study approved by the National Cancer Institute. She described the differences between the standard treatment and the research study, then said we had time to decide—she would leave us a description of the two treatments along with the consent form for the research study. Basically, the standard treatment involved seven weeks of radiation (34 treatments) that she would direct, accompanied by a year of chemotherapy which Dr. Binder would oversee (a chemotherapy drug called BCNU administered every eight weeks). The research study, on the other hand, would add a second drug, cisplatin, and the radiation would start after the first three months of chemotherapy. The research study also required periodic stays in the hospital of several days' duration. "We do not know which of these treatments is better," she said, a statement I later found repeated in the literature.

After Dr. Pierce left, I held Diana in my arms. We did not cry. We hurt. My head swirled with the complexity of the choice. She already had had the surgery, so we were looking at her living another four to six months, and as the tumor grew back, she would have more and more seizures. If we chose to follow the surgery with a standard treatment of radiation and chemotherapy to slow the return of the tumor, we had one-to-three years. If we chose the surgery plus the research treatment, we were in unknown territory but probably had the same chance of one-to-three years. Doctors Dennis, Binder, and Pierce all believed in an aggressive treatment. To us, however, the standard five treatments of radiation per week for seven weeks, plus six treatments of chemotherapy beginning on the first day of radiation and repeating every eight weeks seemed aggressive, if not brutal. Diana and I knew we had several days to make a choice about treatment, but we also knew we didn't have much choice if we wanted to prolong her life. The kicker was the great unknown—the quality of life. Any of the horrible things Dr. Pierce rattled off could happen to Diana, but I so wanted her to live that I had trouble accepting the possibility that we might some day wish we had chosen an earlier death.

Over the weekend, we talked to John, reading and re-reading the literature describing in detail the differences between the standard and research treatments. In the end, we chose the standard treatment because the chances of the research study being more effective seemed marginal. And we chose radiation and chemotherapy over no treatment at all because we thought we had a chance of prolonging her life.

Within days they removed the bandages, and the scar was unnoticeable because her hair fell over the small swath Dr. Dennis had shaved above her right temple. Her olive complexion had a depth of tone, and the lines of her face were gentle. She once again looked good.

Eight days after the surgery, Dr. Dennis checked her eyes and the strength in her hands to determine if there were any signs of weakness. There were none. The surgery had left no noticeable side effects. John took Diana for a walk around Crocket Park on Saturday, and she told him, "I feel like my old self." The next day, she walked down the path in our back yard looking at the red impatience border she had planted in the spring. She later recalled this walk as the last time she felt normal.

I took Diana in to Fairfax Hospital for a CAT scan at 10:30 a.m. on November 5th 1996. John had returned to Kentucky, and I felt the singular weight of responsibility. I had to remind myself that if I screwed up, she might die. Then another voice said, "She's going to die anyway. Relax. Do your best and let go of the rest."

I had read the pamphlets Dr. Pierce had given us about CAT scans, radiation, and chemotherapy, then discussed them with John. As I understood it, a CAT (Computerized Axial

Tomography) scan combines an X-ray and a computer to take a picture of the brain, and Diana needed a CAT scan to determine the points in her brain where the radiologists were to direct the radiation. They couldn't use the MRI photos she had taken on October 18th because the brain had shifted once Dr. Dennis removed the tumor. Diana and I had once gone to a French restaurant in Warrenton where the waitress said the chef had prepared in a particularly delicious sauce to accompany lamb's brain, and when she asked me if that's what I wanted, like a seven-year old with a frog in his pocket, I said, "Why not." It was indeed delicious, but it also was soft like jello, and oozie like mucous. Because of this experience, it was easy to imagine Diana's tumor pushing her mushy brain against her corpus callosum, and, once the tumor was removed, the mushy brain oozing back to fill the empty space. In addition, as John pointed out to me, they couldn't use an MRI just in case Dr. Dennis left a piece of metal in Diana's brain. The magnets in the MRI would pull the metal toward itself, slicing through the brain.

    The pamphlets pointed out that the radiologist had to position the patient on the radiation table very precisely with a plastic mask over the head and tattoos on the scalp so the computer could target the remnants of the tumor. In other words, even if the MRI had been done the day before, the radiologist still needed her own CAT scan.

    Dr. Pierce led us into a cavernous white room with a large white machine. I stayed with Diana as she lay on the table and as the doctors and technicians described the procedure; it seemed harmless enough, yet I hated being there. Everything was so strange to me, and I knew the CAT scan preceded radiation that I thought of as a treatment that burned. Diana looked brave, but when I held her hand, it felt cold. I was grateful for Dr. Pierce because she understood the emotional side of this terrible disease. When the technicians were ready to begin the CAT scan, they asked me to leave the room, just as they would have asked me to leave an x-ray room.

Diana later described the procedure. They began by submerging a piece of aquaplast or plastic mesh in warm water for about a minute until it became pliable, then placed it on her face, pulled it around her head, and anchored it on the head rest. With their fingers, they molded it to the contours of her face and scalp. Diana asked them to cut out the hole for her nose to make her breathing more comfortable. To make sure the mask would be positioned correctly each time she had a radiation treatment, they made small tattoos on her scalp with India ink and a needle (the needle pricks allowed the ink to penetrate the skin). It was similar to a commercial tattoo. I later saw these tiny "cross-hairs" and thought them cute. The CAT scan machine then took pictures of her brain much like slices in a loaf of bread, and the computer then put these X-rays back together to form a three-dimensional picture. Later the radiologists went through each slide to map out the areas of the brain where they would direct the radiation. They also went through a dry run of a treatment to make sure there weren't any mistakes.

They ended by feeding Diana's program for radiation treatments into the computer so that no one else could receive her treatments by mistake. The radiologists also prepared lead shields to be placed on her face and scalp, thus allowing the radiation to hit only the intended areas.

We left the hospital with the first of 34 radiation treatments scheduled for Wednesday, November 13, 1996, and the last to occur on January 2, 1997, every weekday except Thanksgiving and the day after.

I grew to dread the five-day-a-week drive to Fairfax Hospital for radiation. Even though it was only 45 minutes, half of it along a comfortable interstate after the morning rush hour, I felt like I was driving Diana to her death. I just knew the radiation was frying her brain, and I found it increasingly difficult to look beyond the side effects to the long-term benefits. With each successive treatment, she grew weaker and weaker. It was almost a game—how close can we take her to death's door without killing her?

The terribleness of it all also got to Diana. John had come home for several days in early December to give us a hand. He was driving us back from the hospital when Diana began to sob. She sounded like a mother crying over a dead child. John asked her if he should pull off the road, but she couldn't stop crying to answer. I told John to continue, that she had enough strength to make it home. John later explained that the pain, frustration, disappointment, and anger were getting to her at the same time the radiation was frying the emotional centers of her brain.

Parking in the parking garage at Fairfax Hospital is free for oncology patients. On most days, as far as I was concerned, this was the only good thing about radiation. We parked in the oncology section, and in November, Diana was strong enough to walk across the walkway, ride the elevator down two stories, walk into the hospital, and ride another elevator down one floor to radiation. In December, as she weakened, I would park outside the lobby of the hospital, walk her in to sit in one of chairs, and check to make sure she was strong enough to sit there by herself. Then I would park the car in the parking garage, race down to the radiation unit, grab a wheel chair, and wheel it up to the lobby. Finally, I would help her into the wheel chair and roll her down to radiation. Of course, leaving radiation was the reverse process. It was harrowing; whenever I was away from her, I worried that she might have a seizure or collapse. I raced back and forth to keep her in sight.

Once we reached the radiation unit, we would sit in the reception area. We talked quietly, or I read to her from magazines stacked on the end tables. Within ten minutes, they called us over the speaker to go back to another waiting area known as the deck because it was slightly raised. After another five minutes, they called, "Mrs. Gallehr," and she walked or rode the wheel chair back to the radiation room. There she laid on the table as they placed the plastic mask on her head and positioned the lead shields. Once in place, I and the technicians left the room, closing the vault-like lead door behind us. I went back to the deck to read student papers or magazines. The technicians stood in front of a console of dials, looking like pilots of a space ship. Within minutes, they were finished and Diana returned to the nurses' station.

On Wednesdays, the nurses weighed her, on Thursdays, we met with Dr. Pierce, and on Mondays, Tuesdays, and Fridays we asked the nurses questions whenever we needed help. One day Janet, one of the nurses, came up to me and complimented me on bringing Diana to radiation. I was surprised. It was obvious that Diana couldn't make it on her own—someone had to bring her—and we were in this together. We had promised to stick it out "for better or worse," and this, unfortunately, was the "worse."

Then Janet said, "A lot of husbands don't, you know."

"What do you mean?" I asked.

"A lot of husbands leave their wives when they get cancer. They can't take it."

I have since met women whose husbands did just that.

The side effects of the radiation were severe. In the beginning, Diana walked from the car to the radiation unit. By the end, we were lucky to make it in a wheel chair. By early December, she had trouble sitting up without her head leaning to the left because the surgery and radiation to the right hemisphere had weakened her left side. Dr. Dennis approved physical therapy treatments to stretch out the painful knots that developed in her left shoulder. By her sixth radiation treatment, she was spitting up, and Dr. Dennis prescribed Zofran, a drug that controls nausea. In addition, Diana continued to have seizures from time to time despite Dilantin. At her 12th treatment, she had such a strong seizure in the hospital that Dr. Azaam prescribed an additional anti-seizure medication, Tegretol. By 30th treatment at the end of December 1996, she had become incontinent twice.

After radiation, she lost hair on both sides of her head. It was like beating an elephant until it drops to its knees.

Each Wednesday, Diana stood on the scale in the radiation unit to weigh herself. Because radiation tends to destroy your appetite and make you weak, sometimes too weak to eat, the nurses wanted to make sure she wasn't losing too much weight. She lost about ten pounds in the first several weeks, and when she dipped lower, we increased the fat in her diet.

The scale, however, proved to be another measure of her deterioration. In the beginning of radiation, she was strong enough to step up on the scale by herself. As she grew weaker, it was harder and harder for her to lift her feet the necessary five inches. Near the end of her treatment, she was too weak to weigh herself, and we skipped it. Neither Diana nor I became outwardly upset that she could not weigh herself, but inside I was very sad. Diana never talked about it.

We will never know the effect of the radiation on Diana's tumor because we never had a second MRI. The reason for a second MRI would have been to satisfy our curiosity about the condition of the tumor or map the brain for further radiation. None of us, Diana, the doctors, nor I, wanted another MRI. In addition, because Diana received full-brain radiation, only a few more treatments would have been permitted, and that amount would have been insufficient to stop the progress of the tumor. Based on her ability to recover, my guess was that the radiation, along with the surgery and chemotherapy, did a significant job of eradicating the bulk of the tumor. We knew all along that the tumor was like a spider web and that it would grow back if not completely removed. We also knew that it was impossible to completely remove all the little tentacles. We just hoped it would give her an additional year.

Chemo

The day after surgery, Dr. Binder gave us written material from the Eastern Cooperative Oncology Group that compared the standard treatment of radiation and chemotherapy with the clinical trials. This material was more scientific and more blunt about the prognosis than the pamphlets and booklets provided by Fairfax Hospital and various cancer organizations. For instance, "Patients with malignant primary brain tumors have a poor prognosis. Adults with glioblastoma multiforme have a median survival of 8 to 10 months from the time of diagnosis when treated with standard radiation therapy and chemotherapy." This prognosis was shorter than the one to three years Dr. Binder had stated, and I wondered if this were a fact or if they stressed the inefficiency of the standard treatment to persuade us to choose the clinical trials.

Another sentence in this material was sobering because it spelled out the incurable nature of glioblastoma multiforma: "Radiation therapy clearly improves survival, but because it is unable to completely eradicate all tumor cells, recurrent disease is a principal problem." In the back of our minds, we knew the cancer would return, but we were trying to figure out how to get rid of as much of the tumor as possible in order to buy enough time to be eligible for any new treatments, such as gene therapy, that might work.

We knew that chemotherapy was successful in treating some cancers, such as breast cancer, but we learned only when reading about brain cancer that the brain has a barrier called the blood-brain barrier that prevents poisons, including chemotherapy drugs, from entering the brain. In treatments where they penetrated the barrier, the brain was poisoned. This particular clinical trial wanted to compare survival time with a new chemical, and nowhere in the literature was there mention of the new chemical being effective in curing the disease.

It was clear that chemotherapy did not have a track record with Diana's form of brain cancer. I will never forget Dr. Binder's statement that whatever decision we made would be the right one. In other words, even forgoing chemotherapy would be right. I refused to acknowledge that the treatment might kill her.

The whole concept of purposely putting poison into our bodies was foreign to us. We had been careful to eat food that was, if not free of herbicides and pesticides, at least food that was good for us. For the most part, we avoided junk food, and neither of us smoked. We tried to use natural fertilizers on the lawn, and even tried natural remedies for fleas on the pets. Remaining healthy for us was a matter of avoiding poison in its many forms. After reading the literature and talking with John, Brendan, and Marisa, we chose chemotherapy with considerable reluctance, and only to buy time.

Diana's first radiation treatment was at 12:45 p.m. on Wednesday, November 13, 1996. Her first chemotherapy was at 3:00 p.m. that same afternoon. We waited for a short period in the large, L-shaped waiting room with as many as 15 patients—some waiting to receive chemotherapy, as we were, some waiting for the results of blood tests, and others waiting to be examined by one of the oncologists. The place had the feel of a railroad station with passengers waiting to board trains. A number of patients were alone, while others were with loved ones. The conversations were hushed, and nurses interrupted as they called out the last names of patients who struggled to stand, only to amble through the doors and disappear into the interior.

When our turn came, the nurse called our name and ushered us down a long corridor to the chemotherapy room that had large windows, a nurse's station, a television, and comfortable chairs for patients. She then asked us a series of questions, and Diana presented her left arm. The nurse hooked up a bag of chemotherapy much like an IV, and adjusted the flow. She said it would take about an hour, and if the burning sensation at the point of insertion became uncomfortable, she would slow it down.

I had brought along student papers and read them to Diana to pass the time. She was calm. Diana and Marisa had listened to relaxation tapes loaned to us by my friend and colleague Bob Karlson who described the chemicals as beneficial. Because I had been so busy with other things, I had never listened to them myself, and I can only imagine that Diana recalled the tapes as the chemo dripped into her body. We chatted, making up conversation, and when the burning increased, the nurse slowed the drip. At the end of the treatment, the nurse removed the needle and placed a simple bandage on Diana's arm.

As we drove home that evening, we were emotionally exhausted.

Our weekly return visits to the lab situated just off the waiting room were also stressful. The chemotherapy unit and lab were about a quarter mile beyond the radiation unit, so we had to drive from one to the other. We were scheduled for blood work on Mondays after radiation, and as Diana became weaker, the visits to the lab became more difficult. I eventually had to use a wheel chair to get her in and out of the lab.

Her second chemo treatment was scheduled for eight weeks after her first, on Wednesday, January 8, 1997. We had a 10:30 a.m. appointment with Dr. Binder to make sure she was strong enough. Soon after we entered the examination room, Diana felt so weak that she had to lie down on the table. When Dr. Binder came in, she sat up. He listened to her heart, checked her reflexes and strength, and looked at the retinas of her eyes. Instead of saying she was fine, he made a non-committal sound, and I thought he sensed that something was not right, but he didn't say anything, and I didn't ask. I didn't want him to tell Diana that he found something alarming. He then looked at the lab results and said she was OK. I was surprised. I would have delayed the chemo treatment until she felt stronger. The only thing I can conclude is that he was acting on our expressed interest in treating this disease aggressively, even if it threatened her life. It didn't matter that she was extremely weak.

We sat in the same room for the second treatment. It was January, and I had no student papers to read. We saw a young man come in, sit in a chair, stick out his arm, and receive his chemo treatment while watching television. He looked like he was sitting in a car dealership, waiting for a salesman.

I turned to Diana. She looked as if sitting in the chair were taking all her strength. Her head was leaning to the right as she looked up at me with the sweetest eyes. We talked, and I tried to make her comfortable. I felt so, so sorry for her that she had to suffer so much. I felt us growing closer and closer as we traveled further and further from normalcy.

Several weeks later, January 17, 1997, we had an appointment with our neurosurgeon, Dr. Dennis, in Reston. It lay about 30 miles from home and took an hour. It was at a time when Diana was very weak and the weather was cold and windy. It was a herculean effort for her to muster the energy to get up, get into the car, and get there without a seizure. She did not have the strength to walk from the parking lot to the medical building, so I drove up to the door, walked her up to the fourth floor, and made sure she could sit up on the large foyer sofa while I parked the car. When I made it back to her, she had to use the ladies room, so I waited outside with the door propped open. I was afraid that she might pass out and hit her head on the commode or the floor. When she staggered out, I was relieved and happy, and we proceeded to amble down the hall to Dr. Dennis's door.

I turned the doorknob, but it did not budge. I looked to make sure we had the right door. I knew Diana could not stand up much longer, so we turned around and walked back to the foyer. I was sure I had not made a mistake, sure I had copied down the right date. I took out our black schedule book John had bought us after her first seizure, and checked it twice. I was correct. I was angry. I had persuaded Diana that this was an important appointment and that we had to keep it. Seeing the neurosurgeon at the specified intervals would allow us to ask questions and to have him check her. I made sure Diana was OK to leave for a minute, then walked over to the pay phone and called Dr. Dennis's Washington office. The receptionist said, "Oh, he's in Egypt on vacation." No apology. Someone had forgotten to call us. I made another appointment, walked back to Diana, and said, "He's in Egypt on vacation."

"Egypt?" she said. Her voice carried an endearing mixture of surprise, amazement, wonder, and incredulity, without one drop of annoyance or anger. She was usually not riled by such things, but this reaction was different. It was sweet.

I walked her down to the first floor, made sure she was secure sitting on the sofa in the foyer, fetched the car, ran in, and walked her out into the cold, cold, wind. She dozed on the way home, declining my offer to stop anywhere she liked, including visiting her office or her friend Kitty.

I felt so sad watching this woman who, only three months earlier, was strong and capable. Ironically, she was now the sweetest I had ever known her—almost angelic. I can still hear her say, "Egypt?"

In January, 1997, I began to help her wash and bathe because she was so weak. One morning, rather than have her walk to the bathroom, I had her sit on the side of the bed, washed her face with a wash cloth, dabbed on facial lotion, and rubbed it in. When I finished, she took the bottle, poured lotion on her fingers, and rubbed it on my face. I sat there smiling, happy as a four year old.

Despite our arguing throughout our marriage about making love, the actual lovemaking was always very good. When she became ill, I lost all desire to make love. In my mind, making love is two people actively involved in using their bodies to produce love. If it's to get sexual pleasure, it's sex. There were times when selfishness tripped us into sex, but for the most part we made love.

Some time in November 1996, we tried to make love. I thought Diana was strong enough, and I thought it might give her some comfort. Unfortunately, it didn't work because she ran out of energy. She was willing to be passive, but I couldn't see her getting anything out of it, and I felt as if I were taking advantage of her. So we stopped, and I held her in my arms. I wanted her to know that it was OK with me that we stopped. Before I could say anything, she said in a sweet, sweet voice, "It's OK. We'll make love when I'm better."

"Yes," I said, and rocked her back and forth.

I'll never know if she thought it was going to be the last time we would make love, but in my heart, I knew.

A few months later, while taking a bath, she played in the tub like a child, moving the water back and forth with her hands, rubbing the wash cloth along her arms with a sense of wonder. I was fascinated, and couldn't take my eyes off her. Then she looked up at me with the face of a child, the water dripping down her neck, her eyes open and guileless, her mouth innocent and happy.

Much later, when I asked John what might have caused this childlike behavior, he said it might have come from stress, such as the soldier in the foxhole crying for his mommy, but more likely, it came from the chemo damaging the higher inhibited thoughts in the brain. How ironic that the "cure" for the disease was also "curing" our relationship.

First Openings

Diana's illness was the catalyst for our moving beyond our life-long habits, and two events stand out in my mind as instrumental in our opening up to each other, both occurring in late November of 1996. Diana's radiation treatments were scheduled for 10:00 a.m. at Fairfax Hospital, some 30 miles away, which meant we had to leave the house by 8:45. I never liked being late, and Diana knew it. I would often be ready to leave for a party well in advance of the time we were due, then seethed when she would take her time getting ready. Even when relatives visited, she moved at her own pace and would not be hurried. Of course, my becoming angry when she was late played into her half of the dynamic. In the beginning of our marriage, I don't think I told her how important it was for me to be on time. Later, when I did, I felt as if she summarily dismissed my wishes.

As the radiation treatments continued through November, it took Diana longer and longer to get ready in the mornings. She dawdled in the bathroom, taking long showers, then once she made it down to the kitchen, she called her voice mail rather than eat breakfast. In the end, she was late, and I was angry. We were arriving at 10:15 a.m. for our 10:00 a.m. appointments, and eventually the nurses asked us to be prompt because it backed up other patients.

One morning, as we drove along Route 66 toward Fairfax Hospital, I told Diana I didn't like being late. My words were not harsh, but the tone was unmistakable—cold, hard anger. She didn't say anything, so I looked over at her. She was crying, and then she vomited. The radiation and chemotherapy had made her so weak that she was unable to take being upset. I gave her a towel we had in the car in case she got sick, and she wiped her lips and chin. I had never before seen the effect of my anger on her, and it broke my heart. It was the last time I was angry with her.

Several weeks later in one of our visits to Dr. Susan Lord, a doctor specializing in both traditional and alternative medicine, Susan asked us if there were anything we wanted to talk about. I brought up the problem we were having with getting to Fairfax Hospital on time for radiation treatments, and told her I thought Diana was taking her time getting ready. Susan turned to Diana and said, "It sounds like Don is trying his best to get you to the hospital on time. Why are you making it difficult for him?" It was the first time anyone had asked her. Diana was quiet, and I could see that she was thinking it over. After that, she did her best to be on time.

These two events were simple in the large scheme of things, but they were our initial openings to each other. A few months later, I said to her, "It looks like we're opening our hearts to each other," and she agreed.

"Do you think your heart was open before you got sick?"

"No," she said.

Of course, death was both catalyst and a crucible. Knowing the prognosis was one-to-three years made us aware that we had very little time. Diana's life, as well as our life together as a couple, was coming to a close.

Why?

One day as Dr. Dennis was examining Diana, she asked him if he thought her cancer had been caused by her hitting her head on a joist on the way down to our basement, something she had done earlier in the year. "No," he said. "I don't think so." But when we asked him what did cause it, he said he didn't know. Of course, he wasn't the only one we asked. We asked our other doctors, we looked for clues in the literature on brain cancer, and we tried to piece together information we knew about our lifestyle and Diana's relatives.

Diana seemed less driven by looking for an answer than I. I hated the void of not knowing. In education, you get praise, acceptance, awards, honors, and money for knowing. If you don't know, you find out. You do the research, you do the interviews, and you make connections and figure it out. So, in the dark hours of the night and the quiet times driving back and forth to the hospital, in those countless times of walking down the stairs or turning the wheel into the parking lot, in those moments when I didn't have to think, I asked, "Why?"

And rather than sitting with my old nemesis, Doubt, I tried out one answer after another.

First, I blamed myself. I did it. I gave her cancer. If only I had been a better husband, she would be healthy. If only I had not been angry at her, if only I had been happy in the marriage, if only I had taken care of my end of the relationship, she would be well. Everyone knows that unhappiness can lead to illness. I made her unhappy, her immune system dropped, and she caught cancer, much like catching a cold.

I recalled our wedding and the moment her father placed her hand in mine. If I had had any idea then that Diana would have come down with brain cancer when she was 54, I would have taken much better care of her, or so I thought, but only after the fact.

I was not happy with our marriage. I felt cold when I was around her. I wanted her to be warm, to open up her heart, to drop the cerebral, to become close. I knew when I felt warm. I felt warm around my cat. I felt warm around our friends. I pointed out women who made me feel warm. "See Stephanie. She makes me feel warm. Why can't you be like her?"

It didn't matter that there were moments when she did open up, because when she did, it was such strange territory that it scared the hell out of me. I was also afraid that at any moment the arctic winds of fact and logic would storm through and leave me shivering. I couldn't get warm enough for long enough to trust her to place my emotions first.

Then I blamed her cancer on her overall unhappiness. Granted, I don't know how happy she was on the happiness index because she was a very, very private person. As with many people, there were times when I think she dulled her unhappiness with a few too many glasses of wine, and I wondered if the alcohol had broken through the blood-brain barrier and poisoned her brain. She didn't drink a lot, maybe three glasses of wine during a short dinner, but I still urged her to drink less, to limit herself. When I talked to her this, she did not respond, and I felt powerless. I tried replacing some of the wine in the bottle with water, and if anything, I think she drank more. Of course this is understandable if she were drinking to numb the feeling of unhappiness. Then, one night out of desperation, I gave a demonstration. I poured a glass of wine to overflowing, spilling it over the table and onto the floor. "You're destroying our relationship with your drinking," I said. Diana continued to cook dinner as if I were not there. I thought she might be getting some perverse pleasure out of getting me angry, or even of keeping my attention on her. I do know that nothing changed.

I blamed her cancer on the stress of her job. She was manager of the billing division of a large international phone company, billing business customers (as opposed to residential customers) throughout North America. Some customers had monthly phone bills measuring five inches thick. She was on call 24 hours a day, and sometimes, when the computers balked at processing hundreds of thousands of calls for each billing cycle, she got calls in the middle of the night. Even though she rarely brought work home, stayed late, or worked weekends, she drove a very stressful hour in the morning and an hour again in the evening along Route 66 through fast and congested traffic.

I blamed her bosses. She reduced the billing cycles from three days to one, she delighted the people working with and under her, she even went out of her way to take courses and pursue advanced degrees, yet her bosses treated her department as a stepchild, blaming it for problems it did not create, and depriving it of adequate resources to keep her best employees from drifting into other divisions.

Through several conversations with John, it became clear to me that chances were that none of these had caused her cancer. John said, "Stress may or may not have been a contributing factor, but at present, there is inadequate research to say, and if stress had caused a dip in her immune system, she would have suffered colds and the flu before getting cancer." As I said earlier, she was healthy—no colds, flu, or illness of any kind.

At another point, John said, "Recent studies show that lifestyle is a major cause of cancer." For instance, smoking, drinking, sunbathing, eating charcoal-burned food, or being exposed to radioactive substances can cause cancer, but you have to do these things in significantly large doses.

"Alcohol was probably not a factor because there is no evidence from the medical community that it causes brain cancer." Only after John said this did it occur to me to link alcoholics with brain cancer victims. I had never heard of any such connection, and Diana was certainly not an alcoholic. Furthermore, if she were to get cancer from heavy drinking, it would have shown up as liver or stomach cancer, just as heavy smoking leads to lung cancer, heavy sunbathing leads to melanoma, and so forth.

"It is possible that her cancer was genetic," John said. "We're born with cancer suppressor genes, and if you have all of them, you don't get cancer. If you have some of them, you get cancer when you're old. If you have none of them, you get it when you're young. Of course there are other genes that also play a role in getting cancer, and if you have the unlucky combination, you get it."

Her family had a history of cancer—both her mother and aunt died of cancer, as did several of her cousins, although to my knowledge, none of them had brain cancer. Genes can dispose a person to cancer in general, or a particular type of cancer, so it is possible that her "unlucky combination" had been set since birth. Because the tumor Dr. Dennis removed is sitting on a shelf in some warehouse, we may some day be able to check the genes and know for sure.

In the first months of her illness, I desperately wanted to know why Diana got brain cancer. Ever so slowly, time wore away my asking, until I accepted not knowing, and filled my days with taking care of her.

Testing Alternatives

Reiki—Hands on Healing

In 1988, the Northern Virginia Writing Project invited an art therapist from the public schools to give a workshop us writing teachers about art therapy and writing. At one point in the workshop, she asked us to draw a picture, so I drew something with two golden balls hanging from a string that swung back and forth. I didn't know what it meant, and as far as I was concerned, it was just a drawing.

When the art therapist looked at it, she said, "You're going to become involved in hands-on healing."

I turned to her and said, "You're out of your mind."

It was not like me to be so blunt, but her prediction was so far from my experience that I could not imagine it.

A year later, I was sitting in a Reiki I class, training to be a hands-on healer.

A Reiki treatment by a Reiki practitioner consists of gently placing hands on the client in a series of positions, from head to toe, skipping the breasts and genitals to avoid arousal. Even though the client is fully clothed, the client can feel the heat from the practitioner's hands. I know from receiving Reiki treatments from Reiki teachers and Reiki classmates, as well as from myself, that my body relaxes in response to the touch and the warmth of the treatment. I believe that this deep relaxation boosts the immune system and thereby promotes healing. A typical treatment takes about 75 minutes.

I have always loved touch, but before 1989, I had had no contact with alternative medicine or the healing arts. I really liked the Reiki I class, and followed it by taking a Reiki II, the intermediate level of training.

Before Diana's illness, I gave Reiki treatments to about a dozen people, only upon request. Unlike a few of my classmates, I was not interested in it as a business or profession, but rather as a way to keep myself healthy and to help the few people who came to me. I never advertised, charged, or accepted payment.

I can give one example of the effect of Reiki. It was the day of Brendan and Tracy's wedding. We had just finished the pre-wedding photos when one of the bridesmaids said she had a horrible headache.

"Would you like me to do something about it," I asked her.

"Yes," she said.

I placed my hand on her head for about a minute while everyone in the wedding party watched. She was quiet for that minute, and at the end of it, her headache was gone. John's explanation for this is that the headache was caused by tension in her scalp muscles, and the relaxation of those muscles dispersed the pain.

Other clients have mentioned that they felt a weight lifted from them as a result of the treatments. Again, I attribute this to deep relaxation.

When Diana became ill, I thought Reiki might help her to, if not fight the cancer, at least extend and improve the quality of her life. Traditional medicine had given us a horrible prognosis, and I wanted something better. I had known only one Reiki master, Marta Getty, the woman who had given me my Reiki training, and she had told stories of patients with varying ailments who had improved. As far as I was concerned, that was enough.

Finished Business

Diana was skeptical about Reiki, and, in the seven years since my Reiki training, had never requested a treatment. When she became sick, I offered to give her Reiki treatments. She said she thought they would do no harm and they might even help. This was the same statement that traditional medicine made. Because I wanted Diana to receive the most powerful Reiki treatments I could offer, soon after her surgery I met with another Reiki Master (Marta Getty had moved to Europe), explained my situation, and received the training necessary to become a Reiki Master myself.

Before giving Diana her first treatment, I wondered if I should treat her head because if Reiki promoted healing and growth of cells, it might also promote the growth of cancer cells. I also wondered if it might interfere with the radiation. Dr. Susan Pierce, our radiation oncologist, said she had never heard of Reiki, but that she saw no harm in it as long as I did not place heat against Diana's head. My Reiki master also did not know what effect the Reiki treatments might have on Diana's brain or the radiation. She advised me to trust my intuition. Unfortunately, my intuition on this subject was weak. In the end, I decided not to treat her head. I will never know if this was a wise decision.

I gave Diana her first Reiki treatment on November 7, 1996, about a week before she began radiation. In our guest room, I set up the massage table we had, placed a boom box on the coffee table, and played Richard Wagner's "Quiet Heart," a soothing tape of flute music. Diana laid on her back on the massage table. I placed a down pillow under her knees and another under her head. I then covered her with a grey, Belgian flannel sheet.

"How is that?" I asked her.

"Comfortable," she said.

I began by running my fingers through her hair, gentle movements to put her at ease. Mentally, I said a prayer asking that only good come to Diana from this treatment. I then placed my cupped hands over her closed eyes, allowing energy and warmth from the palms of my hands to warm her eyes and cheeks. She was quiet. I could hear her breathing lengthen. I watched her chest rise and fall—she was breathing deeper, almost sighing. After about five minutes, I moved my hands over her ears, and I could feel them become warm. After another five minutes, I moved down to her clavicle and so on down the front of her body. She chose not to talk, but I knew she had not fallen asleep. When I reached her feet, I added a gentle massage, then asked her to turn over. As she did, I removed the pillows, then began the treatment again on her shoulders and moved down her back. At the end of the treatment, I placed one hand on the back of her neck and the other on her sacrum, then gently rocked her back and forth. I lifted my hands as quietly as I could, stepped away from the table, and sat in the wing chair.

After a few minutes, she sat up. "That was nice," she said. She was calm and sweet, much like a small child waking from a satisfying sleep.

"Thank you," I said. I was relieved that she liked it.

"Very nice," she added. Her response made me very happy.

As she proceeded through radiation treatments in November and December, she grew very weak, and before long, she was unable to turn over during a Reiki treatment without seizing, so I treated her front, then slid my hands beneath her to treat her back. Eventually, in January of 1997, she became so weak she would fall asleep soon after supper. When I asked her if she would like a Reiki treatment, she would say, "Not tonight—I'm a little tired." I felt so sorry for her.

I gave Diana Reiki treatments throughout her illness, although not always full treatments nor treatments every day. I think the treatments were relaxing for her, and I believe they contributed, perhaps in some small way, to her health. I think they also gave her a sense of my physical love for her.

People have asked me what impact did my giving her these treatments have on me, and I've said that I found them to be both powerful and soothing. I liked the physical sensation of energy passing through my hands, and I liked the idea that I was able to do something for her during a period when I felt powerless against the much larger forces of the cancer.

Nutrition

Several years after we were married, Diana had a severely ruptured eardrum, and her doctor scheduled her for surgery. In the meanwhile, she had heard of the benefits of vitamin A for healing the ear, and proceeded to take the dosages recommended. When she returned to the doctor two weeks later, he looked into her ear and apologized for getting the wrong ear. When he looked into the other one, he realized that the ruptured eardrum had healed.

Over the years, Diana took vitamins every day, and I think she was healthy in part due to the vitamins. She regularly took—in separate capsules, vitamins A, C, and E and Folic Acid, varying the amounts according to her current health. For instance, when she felt a cold coming on, she took more vitamin C.

When she got cancer, we looked for a doctor versed in alternative medicine and nutrition and found Dr. Susan Lord who practiced in Washington. Susan was an attractive, warm, and caring physician with a soothing voice who did as much for our emotional health as she did for Diana's physical health.

We told Susan that we were interested in nutrition that would help fight the cancer and detoxify the body from the drugs and treatments. Susan loaned us a video tape about Anne Frahm who had recovered from breast cancer after it had spread to her shoulder, ribs, skull, pelvic bone, and vertebrae. After going through a horrendous series of surgery, radiation, and chemotherapy treatments from which she almost died, Anne looked like death. We bought the companion book, *A Cancer Battle Plan: Six Strategies for Beating Cancer from a Recovered "Hopeless Case"* which told the story of Anne's search for a connection between cancer and nutrition. Anne had been released from the hospital because the doctors could do no more for her. Once home, she implemented her nutrition program, and within five weeks, she was free of cancer. We were impressed because Anne looked strikingly beautiful and healthy.

We told Dr. Lord that we wanted to try everything that held out hope. Susan recommended a program similar to Anne Frahm's, one aimed at detoxifying the body through a diet of low fat and a regimen of vitamins and nutritional supplements. These were the supplements Diana took.

- Vitamin A
- Vitamin B-Complex
- Beta Carotene
- Vitamin C
- Vitamin E
- Folic Acid
- Selenium
- Copper
- Zinc
- Evening Primrose
- Manganese
- Flaxseed Oil

We took this list to Dr. Pierce, our radiation oncologist, who said that she could see no harm in taking them, except for vitamin E that she limited to 400 I.U. per day because it might interfere with the radiation treatments.

After several weeks on the vitamins and low-fat diet, and after several weeks of radiation, Diana began to lose weight and became weak. I called a toll-free number to talk to Anne Frahm about the advisability of using her detoxification program and diet during radiation only to find that the number was no longer in service. Diana said, "That's not good news." I learned much later that Anne died on February 5, 1998 from the cancer that had returned and spread to her backbone and lungs.

We then checked with Dr. Lord and Dr. Pierce, and followed their advice to increase the fat in Diana's diet, to feed her meat, and to give her milk shakes.

It is worth noting that during this same period we also tried an herbal tea, which was touted in Canada as an anti-cancer agent. We discontinued it when we saw no benefit in drinking it, nor could we find corroborating evidence from the traditional medical community or attention from the media.

John told us that cancer cells are like any other cells, and in 1997, there was no food that fed nor poisoned just cancer cells. In other words, what we fed the body we feed the cancer. We were unable to cure Diana's brain cancer with nutrition, but nutrition and good food did keep her as healthy as possible. She continued to take vitamins throughout her illness, and I believe they helped. It is difficult to say what specific effects these vitamins had on here, but she was not sick once during her bout with cancer.

Energy Work

I have to admit at the outset that I don't understand very much about the energy fields that emanate from the body. I have twice seen my own aura, and once seen someone else's. What I saw was a medium-green light that rose about two inches above my knee and thigh. Each time, I saw it for about a minute, then I couldn't see it any more. In addition, I have seen photos of energy extending from a person's hand, and I once felt the energy of a Zen master push me even though he was about 50 feet away.

So, the bottom line for me is that I know there are such things as energy fields, but I have never been able to manipulate them.

I have two stories to tell about others who could see these energy fields. One person saw my energy field and told me I had some problems with my right foot. She was correct—I had been playing basketball in an old pair of sneakers and had bruised my metatarsal. In fact, it hurt like hell, but she had no way of knowing that. The second story concerns an American Indian who saw the energy field of one of my colleagues and told her that she had problems with her pancreas. This was a year before she was diagnosed with diabetes.

With this as my background, I was receptive to people looking at Diana's energy field, and if there was anything they could do to help her to heal, I was all for it.

The first person was Gerry Eitner who had received training in a procedure she called at the time Christopher Light. Basically, it involved using the fingertips to feel a person's energy field, then if the field showed an imbalance or blockage, correct it through various movements of the hands. When Gerry gave Diana a Christopher Light treatment, Diana sat on the ottoman in our living room, and Gerry moved her hands systematically down Diana's body. The next morning, Diana said to me that she had felt a grey cloud over her for the last few days, but now it was now gone.

Gerry showed me how to do this energy work, but I had difficulty feeling the energy fields, so I did not pursue this form of treatment. All I can say is that some people can sense these fields and work with them, but I'm not one of them.

The other person to help us was Bonnie Ellis, a board-certified massage therapist who had given me several massage treatments over the years. I had great respect for Bonnie, so when Dr. Susan Lord recommended that Diana get a craniosacral massage, I turned to Bonnie. Craniosacral Therapy was developed by Dr. John E. Upledger in the early 1970's to remove the negative effects of stress on the central nervous system, from the top of the head to the tailbone. Therapists can feel an irregularity or obstruction in the rhythm of the craniosacral energy, and with a gentle massage, free up the restriction. I am sure it is much more complex than this, but our simple understanding of it, along with Dr. Lord's recommendation, was sufficient for us to try it.

Bonnie gave Diana only one treatment before Diana became too weak to accept another.

Gene Therapy

I read the early reports from the Brain Cancer Foundation and other sources which indicated that gene therapy was still too experimental to be recommended. I contacted a surgeon in Philadelphia involved in gene therapy, and after my lengthy description of Diana's case, he said that she was not eligible because of her weakened condition. He also said that none of the patients had survived the treatment.

I also talked to our son John and to Eric Maybach, our family physician, about gene therapy, and neither of them could recommend it. The image I was left with was that even if Diana gained enough strength to receive the treatment, she stood a good chance of dying from it—which also meant dying in a hospital. Selfishly, perhaps, I wanted her to be surrounded by those who loved her.

As Diana moved though January and became weaker and weaker, I realized that alternative medicine was no match for the strength of the traditional treatments. Alternative medicine was best as a preventative, but using it in emergency situations was ineffective. Perhaps some day alternative medicine will replace traditional medicine, or that there will be a marriage of the two, but during Diana's illness this was still a long way off. I have to admit that I felt a bit discouraged about the limitations of alternative medicine. Hope was an essential commodity in our daily struggle to beat this cancer, and without it, we were forced to accept the reality of this cancer being a terminal illness.

A Week in the Hospital

The night of Monday, January 27, 1997, Diana spent in and out of a very deep sleep. The next morning, I unsuccessfully tried to wake her to give her meds. I then discovered that she had wet the bed. I didn't know what to do, and I became afraid, knowing I was not prepared to handle this situation. I decided to leave her alone for a few minutes while I raced down to the local drug store to buy Chux Underpads (large square absorbent pads which are placed under a patient), and Depends (diapers for adults). I worried that I might be making a mistake by leaving her alone. What if she had a seizure while I was out of the house? What if she were face down in the pillow when she had a seizure? Would she suffocate? I knew her prognosis was one-to-three years, but I didn't want her to die, and I especially didn't want her to die before her time or because I had left her unattended.

When I returned, she was just as I had left her, and I felt momentarily relieved. I placed a chucks pad beside her hip, rolled her on her side, slid down her wet pajama bottoms, and rolled her further onto her stomach. The movement must have upset something in her head because she vomited, face-down into the bed. When I tried to roll her onto her back to clean her up, I could not. She had become dead weight. I felt horrible—helpless, afraid, and sick.

I called Carol Wickert, a friend of the family who had been staying with Diana while I went to work several days a week during the past few weeks. Carol had been a member of the Warrenton Rescue Squad for many years and had ample experience dealing with emergencies. After I described Diana's condition, she said, "I think you should call your doctor." At this point we had three doctors: our surgeon, Dr. Dennis; our radiation oncologist, Dr. Pierce; and our chemotherapy oncologist, Dr. Binder. Because Diana had finished surgery and radiation, I called Dr. Binder. He was out of the office, so the receptionist transferred my call to one of his colleagues, Dr. Orloff, whom I had never met. After I described Diana's condition, he asked if I could drive her into Fairfax Hospital. I told him she seemed to be unconscious and that we lived in Warrenton, 30 miles away, which meant I would have to call our local rescue squad. I asked him if we could take her to Fauquier Hospital, less than two miles away.

"Yes," he said, so I hung up and called 911.

I heard the sirens almost immediately, and within three minutes, an ambulance pulled up in front of the house. I ran downstairs and opened the front door for two young men who looked like firemen ready to storm a burning building. They wore heavy, black-and-yellow jackets, and black boots. Even though John had run for the rescue squad, and even though I had seen his uniform and boots, I had never seen him on a call. I was impressed at the powerful presence of these men. We rushed upstairs where they immediately checked her pulse and blood pressure, then placed an oxygen mask on her face. They spoke in street voices, asking Diana her name, asking her if she knew what day it was, asking her the name of the president of the United States, and telling her what they were doing. She responded quickly to the oxygen, opened her eyes, and answered their questions. She didn't know what day of the week it was, but she had had trouble with that question ever since surgery. They then placed an IV on her arm in case they had to give her medications before they reached the emergency room. Then the three of us wrapped her in the bed sheet and a large, white rescue squad blanket, slid a board under her, and carried her downstairs to the stretcher standing inside the front door. The two men then rolled her out of the house and into the ambulance.

Driving behind the truck, I felt like a failure because I had been unable to keep her out of the hospital. I had so wanted her to be home, surrounded by family, pets, and the house she loved.

Soon after we arrived in emergency room, the lab technician drew blood and discovered that her Dilantin count was 4.8, considerably below the 10–20 therapeutic range, and her Tegretol count was 2.0, also lower than the therapeutic range of 4–8. The nurse gave her a shot of Solumedrol to reduce swelling in the brain (Salumedrol is easier to administer in shot form than Decadron), and started an IV of 300 milligrams of Dilantin. I was greatly relieved that her loss of consciousness in the morning was nothing more than her drugs being out of whack.

I had called Brendan from the house while waiting for the rescue squad. "Do you want me to come out?" he asked. I hesitated, thinking only in medical terms, thinking that the doctors in the emergency room could handle the situation. I have always been reluctant to have people stand around doing nothing. Brendan knew that, but he was also thinking in human terms. He called Tracy, Marisa, and Glen, and by late morning all of them, plus Carol Wickert who had come based on my call earlier in the morning, were with Diana in the emergency room. I was really glad they were there.

By the afternoon, the emergency room doctor thought Diana should be admitted to the hospital to get her counts under control, and I felt relieved. I did not want a repeat of that morning. Because a patient must be admitted under the care of a physician, he asked us for the name of our doctor. I told him we were currently under the care of three doctors in Fairfax, but that we had no local oncologist. He said Diana could be admitted under the care of our family physician, so we did. Dr. Eric Maybach had been our doctor since moving to Warrenton in 1975, and we also knew him socially, although we had had little regular contact with him over the years because we had been so healthy. The emergency room doctor contacted Dr. Maybach who arranged for a private room for Diana based on her condition. That room became available late in the afternoon.

I knew I would be staying in the room with Diana, helping the nurses take care of her, and sleeping on a chair at night. I would not have left her even if she had been stronger, but knowing she was not able, mentally and physically, to push the call button made it clear to me that it was necessary for someone to be in the room at all times. I knew that if she had to get up to go to the bathroom, I would be there to help her; if she needed a bedside commode, I would help her to sit on it. If she wet the bed, I would call the nurses to change the sheets.

Before going to sleep that night, I ended my journal entry with, "I have to admit, I hate it when she can't remember the day of the week. I want her to be well." Looking back, and considering all she had endured during this day, it seems odd that I was bothered by her inability to remember the day of the week. In my rational mind, I could excuse her because all her days were becoming the same. She no longer went to work, no longer had weekends off. Nevertheless, this one disability was now symbolic of our departure from the normal lives we had lived only a short while ago, lives of health, work, friends, and family.

The next day, Wednesday, January 29, 1997, Randy and Martha (Diana's brother and sister-in-law) arrived from North Carolina to help out. Randy entered Diana's room and, after giving her a hug, said, "How are you? Making sure the interest level stays high?"

On the same day, Dr. Maybach asked me for permission to consult with Dr. Moore, a neurologist whom he greatly respected, and that afternoon I spent a half-hour talking with Dr. Moore.

I showed her the meds book dating back to October 18, with the list of medications and the times Diana took them. She was amazed that I had kept such careful records. I told her that our son, John, had started it, not only to keep track of the medications, but also to make sure I didn't give her the same meds twice, or none at all. I never thought the meds log would serve any other purpose. Dr. Moore tried to see a correlation between seizures and the Dilantin, wanting to get the Dilantin count up to 15, the middle of the therapeutic range. She thought she could achieve that in another day or so. She also increased the Decadron to decrease the headaches.

"Do you know of any new drugs without side effects?" I asked her.

She said there was another form of Dilantin but that it was intravenous and burned, so that was not an option.

She talked about Tegretol and Dilantin competing with each other for binding. As I understand it, both these drugs bind to a protean molecule, and if the Tegretol has already bound to a protean molecule, the Dilantin spills into the body. In an attempt to stop her seizures, two months earlier Dr. Azzam had prescribed Tegretol thinking the Dilantin was not stopping the seizures. Dr. Moore, in another attempt to control the seizures, prescribed Neurontin, a newer drug. Apparently, when seizures are hard to control, doctors have the option to use a higher dosage of one drug or a lower dosage of several drugs. The bottom line was that the seizures had to be brought under control. She also talked about Dr. Dennis, our surgeon, saying that he had performed a very difficult surgery on a patient she knew, a surgery that other doctors would not attempt, and that it was very successful. This was an unsolicited opinion, and I was glad she offered it. I needed to hear that Diana was getting the best help available.

When I asked her about Diana's short-term memory, Dr. Moore said she thought it might be weak for another three to six months. I realized that in the larger scheme of things, that was little enough to suffer. She then said that Dr. Maybach was a cautious man, and she thought he might keep Diana in the hospital until Friday or Saturday. She must have known how eager I was to bring Diana home. When Dr. Moore returned to the room, she asked Diana a number of questions to test her mental abilities, and Diana answered them beautifully.

On Thursday, I taught class, leaving at 11:00 a.m. and returning at 4:00 p.m. Even though Diana was in the hospital and under the care of doctors and nurses, I asked Carol to stay with her while I was away. I didn't want Diana to feel as if she were alone or helpless. When I returned at 4:00 p.m., our daughter-in-law Tracy was also there, so I had time to go home and take a shower.

When I got back to the hospital at 6:00 p.m., Diana was asleep. Tracy said that she had had a few hallucinations, including a dog figurine that disappeared when Diana tried to touch it. This was my first experience with someone who had hallucinations. I knew nothing about them. Later that evening, Dr. Moore explained that Diana's brain was probably firing off in the visual cortex and she was actually seeing something. She also told me that hallucinations are real to the person seeing them.

That evening, I had a half-hour talk with Dr. Maybach and Dr. Moore. Diana's Dilantin count was now 16.0, which meant it was in the therapeutic range. To maintain that level, Dr. Moore thought the Dilantin dosage Diana should be on was about 450 milligrams a day. She also thought that Diana's swings in sprightliness and loss of power might be coming from the brain healing and shedding scar tissue.

When Dr. Moore left, Dr. Maybach said that he thought glioblastoma was a vicious cancer that people did not survive. I was surprised that he was telling me this. I had known since October that there was little chance of anyone surviving this disease. Then it hit me. He was unaware of all we had gone through in the past three months, and also unaware of how much we had learned about this disease. I also thought that he might have read my positive attitude as ignorance. After all, I believed in miracles and would have loved for one to happen to Diana. Nevertheless, there was great sadness in my heart that night.

Saturday, February 1st was Diana's birthday. We had a party in the room with cake, relatives, and friends. Diana sat in a chair, eating her lunch off the bed tray. As she sat there, I watched as her head fell to the right. She seemed engrossed in the meal and didn't have much contact with the rest of us who were pretending to be jovial. I knew that her head flopping to the right had previously been the cause of the knot in her shoulder, but I placed the party as a top priority and let her enjoy it.

The next day, I regretted my not stepping in to hold her head up straight. We were supposed to go home on Sunday, but because her left shoulder was so sore, Dr. Maybach postponed our discharge until Monday. Fortunately, however, Julie Maybach, Dr. Maybach's daughter who was a physical therapist, came into the room to see her father and when she learned that Diana's shoulder was in a knot again, she massaged it until it loosened up.

One of the amazing things I witnessed while Diana was in the hospital one night was her taking her medications. She sat up in the bed and had some difficulty swallowing, so her movements were very slow and purposeful. Diana had me and the two nurses in the room mesmerized as she very carefully moved the pills to her mouth and sipped the juice. This was an activity I was to watch countless times in the year to come, and I was always amazed. Most of us don't pay attention to what we're doing—we eat and talk, or eat and watch television, or eat and read the newspaper. Diana's actions were the very thing the Zen books advocate—doing one thing at a time, mindfully.

During Diana's week in the hospital, I found the nurses, even though they were understaffed and overworked, they were also extremely warm and caring.

Before leaving the hospital to go home, Dr. Maybach said we needed to select a doctor to keep tabs on her. I hesitated to select him because I thought we might need an oncologist, and I didn't know any in Warrenton. When he explained that a family physician was sufficient, I asked him if he would be willing to be our doctor, and he said, "Yes." It was one of the best decisions I made.

Downturn

Even though Dr. Pierce had warned us of the possible side effects of radiation, neither of us was expecting them. As Diana became weaker and weaker, she was increasingly unable to do even the most common of daily activities. My heart went out to her at each downturn, and often at the end of the day, I found myself so sad that I wept.

As the days passed, a larger and larger portion of our time was consumed with doctor's appointments, therapy appointments, managing medications, and simply taking care of the simplest thing in life such as bathing, eating, and moving about. We were surrounding ourselves with health care professionals, nurses, doctors, and physical therapists, and I was surprised that they consistently found something positive to say about Diana's condition even when it was, by our standards, horrible. These people had seen worse, knew the whole picture, and had learned the benefits of stressing the positive.

From the time my parents died in my early 20's, until the time we placed my father-in-law in a nursing home in the early 1990's, I had had very little contact with illness. Not only was our immediate family healthy, our extended family and friends enjoyed good health, too. We visited Diana's father soon after he entered a nursing home, and I was appalled at the deterioration of his fellow patients. Some of them were incontinent, bedridden, almost comatose, or senile (one, a former teacher, cursed in a loud, penetrating voice from morning to night). John said that only a small percentage of Americans end up in nursing homes; nevertheless, the specter of ending up in one, even a good one, like the one my father-in-law lived in for the last five years of his life, was enough to bolster my resolve to do everything I could to keep my loved ones at home.

Because of our long history of being healthy, the first five months of Diana's illness was a huge adjustment for us, and the decline in her condition in November, December, and January was particularly upsetting.

Bob Karlson, a friend and colleague of mine at George Mason, offered to help Diana to cope with the emotional side of cancer. We visited his home, located several miles from Fairfax Hospital, about five times, and it was there that Diana practiced relaxation techniques and listened to tapes prepared specifically for cancer patients. One day in November, Bob invited Diana to use his computer to write about how she felt about her illness. I later found this piece in her pocketbook, and because it does not contain anything I think she would object showing to others, I enter it here exactly as she wrote it. It shows considerable deterioration of her hand-eye coordination, although her thinking seems fine to me.

Dec, 1006 OH damn—I don't really wan ro onccenrate on hi siuation…Hard o lie wh must live with!

Dmn—I houht I was healhthy! Now concer—nd a ad kind not that there are any good kinds. What is so remarkale is ho caring and supportig people have been. It is sourprising how much that means to us. Don has been so wonderful an sweet—kno I couln't do as much if the shoe weree on the other foo. His is scary I'm hoping fo good news after the treatments. Will do th raw foods diet…Especially after readin the Shakle meterial from JO Ann—tht I tocorroorations h it works. Why not? Need to look at work situation too...Jack is a stress factor—or how I deal witthe him is no satisfacory, Has he ever said or done anyhing supporrive fo me or the group in five years? Cn't think of anyhing! Not worth it! Im afraid that ia will have a new tumor anbd have o do this all again. Not for a hile anyway...

Two months earlier, she was writing memos, letters, and proposals for a large international phone company. I didn't say anything to Diana when I found and read this piece, and as far as I know, she was unaware that she was unable to type correctly.

A few months later, during a conversation about her returning to work, Diana tried to use my lap top computer. She became very calm, concentrated on the screen, and typed:

evnjeralfqgvacecqcjr[ocjrgrv

After a few minutes, I said, "I think it best if we try this another time."

"OK" she said. She wasn't at all upset. I was.

One evening, in December 1996, Diana was sitting in our living room watching television. She sat in her favorite place, on our Empire-style sofa that dated back to 1830. Diana's mother had bought this sofa in the 1960's, and the rumor that accompanied it was that Lafayette had slept on it. As I remember it, her mother bought it at auction from one of the fine auction houses in Winchester, Virginia, where Diana's parents lived at the time. Her mother said that the sofa had originally come from a home in Warrenton, Virginia, about 40 miles away, a town Diana and I moved to in 1975. In the 1960's, we had no idea that we would ever live in Warrenton.

Diana and I courted on this sofa. It had a down cushion, which was very comfortable to lounge on, to sleep on, and, of course, to hold hands on. When her parents went upstairs to bed, listening, I'm sure, for sounds from the living room, we, trying to be as quiet as mice, made out on it. When her parents moved to Florida in the early '70's, they gave it to us, and it became the centerpiece of our living room.

Diana loved sitting on it while entertaining guests, while watching *Masterpiece Theater* and PBS shows, and while reading. In the months before she got sick, she would sit on it while I washed the dishes and straightened up the kitchen. Increasingly, she fell asleep on it. I thought she was tired from long days at work, from eating a full dinner, and from the glass of wine she carried with her to the sofa. I had no idea a tumor was growing inside her brain. There were a few times in November and December of 1996, when Brendan noticed that she was sitting on the sofa staring at the television when the channel was 00, and there was nothing on but a blue screen. Diana was never upset when we pointed this out to her. She would always let us change the channel or turn off the television.

That evening in December of 1996, I walked over to her and asked if she were ready to go to bed. She said she was, so I reached my hands under her shoulders and helped her to stand. I then noticed a large, dark maroon stain on the cushion. "I think you've wet the sofa," I said, with gentleness and totally without blame. I think if she had been well, I might have been upset with her, but under the circumstances, I felt so, so sorry for her.

"Oh," she said, looking behind her. She said it with mild surprise, much like one discovering a shiny coin in a parking lot.

"Let's go upstairs, and get you into the tub," I said. I walked beside her up the stairs, helped her peel off her wet slacks and panties, and steadied her as she stepped into the tub. She was very sweet, accepting this mishap in stride. When she was dry and in her pajamas, I tucked her into bed, and kissed her goodnight, much like I had done with our children. I then returned to the living room, unzipped and removed the cushion cover, and dropped it in the washing machine. I laid the cushion out on the back porch, and after a few weeks of fresh air, it had no odor.

That night, as I lay awake in bed beside her, I thought about her incontinence, and it frightened me. She was falling apart. I thought the radiation and chemotherapy would have lessened the cancer, but I did not think it would make her too weak to know she had to visit the bathroom. I wondered what caused her incontinence, and I feared that she might become incontinent on a daily basis. But most of all, I felt so, so sorry for her. I had known her 34 years, and she had never had trouble like this.

After Diana's last radiation treatment on January 2, 1997, we treated ourselves by visiting Picadilly, a fine gift shop in Warrenton. Diana loved shopping at Piccadilly, and enjoyed talking to Charlotte Sedam, the owner. For Diana, Picadilly was a comfort store that restored her spirit as she browsed through the Waterford crystal, the Crabtree and Evelyn bath products, the brass candlesticks that were made in Virginia, the stuffed animals, and the beautiful baby clothes.

Diana was wearing her black, goose-down winter coat, and I was nervous about her walking between the tables of fragile stemware. Several weeks earlier, after taking a nap, she had caught her right foot in the bottom of the bedspread, and had fallen on the floor. She was dazed but otherwise unhurt, and I was relieved that she had not hit her head on the dresser. I was watching her now walk precariously through the narrow aisles of Picadilly before sitting down at the counter. Her dark brown hair was windblown and covered part of her face. She had not had her hair cut in over two months.

Both Charlotte and Diana were tall, elegant, and lady-like, with a taste for fine things. After a few moments of conversation, Charlotte was unable to avoid the obvious. She looked at Diana and said with the utmost kindness, "You don't look particularly well. Have you been sick?"

"Yes, I've had brain cancer," Diana said.

Charlotte's mouth dropped open. This was Diana's first venture into a store in over two months. I had become accustomed to seeing her in physical therapy, radiation, and chemo units, all of which contained people who looked as sick as Diana, and some who looked far worse. Piccadilly, however, was the normal world, the world we once frequented, and the contrast of seeing Diana in such a shaken condition made me enormously sad.

Diana and Charlotte talked for a while about brain cancer, about a friend of Charlotte's who also had brain cancer, and about the treatments. Diana was articulate, using words not usually found in conversation. "All this has not hurt your vocabulary. I'm amazed," said Charlotte.

Diana smiled. I felt very proud of her.

By the middle of January 1997, I knew Diana was growing weaker, but I never knew ahead of time how much. One evening, I prepared her bath and helped her into the tub. "Are you OK to sit up?" I asked her.

She nodded, and I saw her lean back. Ordinarily, she rested in this position, moving the water back and forth across her legs. This time, however, her legs went limp, and she slid under. I reached down, grabbed her arm, and pulled her up. She spit out the soapy water as I unplugged the drain and pressed my hand against her legs until she could lean forward. When the water had completely drained out, I stepped into the tub and lifted her from behind until she could stand. I was so grateful that she had had only a momentary loss of strength because I could not have pulled her out of the tub by myself.

A similar loss of power occurred about this time while John was visiting. Diana and I were upstairs in the bedroom around 9:00 p.m. By now I knew I had to stay close to her, but I didn't have to be in the room with her every single minute. We were heading out of the bedroom, and as we walked down the hall, Diana took a right and entered the bathroom. It was typical of her to wander off without telling me where she was going even when she was healthy, so I didn't think anything of her veering off into the bathroom. I walked down the hall and saw her close the bathroom door, so I figured she had to use the commode. I walked down stairs and waited for her in the living room.

About five minutes later, John came home, said, "Hi," and went upstairs. A few seconds later, he was back down standing in the living room doorway.

"Do you know Mommy's on the floor in the bathroom?" John had opened the door far enough to see her face and to know that she was OK. He thought she might have just stepped out of the shower, and he didn't want to open the door further only to discover his mother naked.

"No," I said. We ran upstairs.

I pushed open the door to find her sprawled across the floor. "Are you alright?" I asked her.

She came to, and we helped her to her feet. Apparently, she had passed out and slumped to the floor, but she had not hurt herself.

One day in January 1997, after returning to Warrenton from Fairfax where we had gone for blood tests, I parked the car in front of the house, walked around to the passenger side, and opened her door to see her sitting with her head leaning on her right shoulder and her hands limp in her lap. "Are you OK?" I asked. "Can you make it into the house?"

"I'm fine," she said. I reached under her arms and tried to help her stand. She was not strong enough, so I helped her to sit back in the passenger seat.

"It's OK. Take your time," I said. "When you're ready, we'll give it another try."

I waited several minutes, glancing up and down the street, hoping someone would come by. No one was on the street, and no cars passed. As far as I could tell, no one was home. I asked her again, "Do you think you can make it?"

"Yes, I'm fine," she said.

I knew she wasn't fine, but I thought she could stand and walk to the house. As I reached under her arms, she pushed herself up and stood. Then she collapsed. I still had my hands under her arms, but I didn't think I could get her safely back into the passenger seat, so I wrapped my arms around her and tried to get my shoulder under her so I could carry her. At six feet tall and close to 140 pounds, she was too heavy for me to sweep up in my arms.

I again looked up and down the street, but saw no one. I didn't want to put her down on the pavement, so I walked backwards toward the gate, dragging her. She was the proverbial dead weight.

I tried to move around behind her so that I could hold her under her arms and half lift, half drag her, but I couldn't. I got inside the gate to the sidewalk when I ran out of strength and rested her down on her shins as gently as I could. With her long legs, it was like trying to hoist a giraffe. I moved around to her back, got my arms under her arms, and dragged her the 18 or so feet to the front porch. I then walked backwards up the two steps and sat down. At this point, I knew she was unconscious, and I laid her on the porch. I was exhausted and frightened. I opened the screen door, propped it open with the door mat, opened the front door, and returned to Diana who looked like a drunk passed out in the gutter, her shirt out of her slacks from my grabbing her under the arms, her midriff exposed.

"OK, we're going to try this again," I told her, but there was no response. From behind her, I pushed her up into a sitting position, slid my arms under her arms, stood, then her, up as far as I could, and dragged her into the living room. Shortly after I laid her on the sofa, resting her head on one end and propping her feet up on the ottoman, she came to.

I called the lab to discover that her Dilantin level was 32 when the therapeutic level was 10–20. She had passed out from too much Dilantin running through her body.

There is a story of a Zen master who is approached by a student wanting instruction. The Zen master takes the student to a barrel of water and pushes his head under, keeping him submerged for a few moments. When he lets him up, he asks the student, "What did you want most when you were under water?"

"Air," the student replied.

The Zen master promptly dismissed the student, saying, "When you want instruction more than air, come back." I don't know that Diana and I wanted intimacy more than air, but we wanted it enough to make it happen.

On January 29, 1997, I wrote in my journal, "Diana is everything I've always wanted in a spouse. It has taken me 31 years to realize that, and I feel so foolish not having known. Maybe it takes 31 years to have this kind of love story. She is still my Zen master—still teaching me wisdom."

On February 1, 1997, I wrote, "Yesterday, while Di was on the porta potty, I was on my knee nuzzling her, and I proposed to her. She accepted. It was funny and cute and loving. She is so cute. The night before she said we were so lucky because we were showing our kids how to take care of each other. This is the best our marriage has ever been. I love her to pieces. We are very sweet to each other. How did we do it? How did we take this trip from a marriage that was on the verge of dissolving to genuine love? I think the cancer and her impending death forced us to open up to each other and let go of our bad habits, and once we did, our love for each other was there."

And on March 11, 1997, I wrote, "I love her so much now that she has opened up. I told her a few days ago, 'All I ever wanted to do was fall in love with you.'"

Heartbreak

Randy and Martha, Diana's brother and sister-in-law, offered to stay with us in Warrenton when we brought Diana home from the hospital in February. I thought she would gain strength because her counts were now in the therapeutic range. Instead, she grew weaker and weaker. In early February, we had to help her to sit up in bed to feed her. Two weeks later, we had to rent a hospital bed for her. It was covered by insurance, and it was absolutely essential if we were to raise and lower her head.

On February 18, 1997, I wrote to Maureen McNulty, an adjunct faculty member at George Mason for whom I served as mentor in the fall of 1996. "I'm sending you this note so that you won't be surprised. Diana is not bouncing back. She is weaker each day. She is now an infant—we change her diaper regularly and rotate her so she doesn't get bedsores. Some days she sleeps a lot, and some days she isn't sure which town she is in. She is still quite beautiful and is teaching us all. The children are gradually learning to let go." I then added, "She will always be with us, but I think in a month or so she will be with us from the spirit world. We went through hell a few weeks ago, but now we're catching some of Diana's serenity."

I think her downturn in February and March of 1997 was a result of the radiation and chemotherapy treatments. Diana once said, "They slash, burn, and poison you, then march you up to death's door." On February 20th, I wrote to Maureen, "Dark days are behind me, and I'm now helping her to die." I had accepted the fact of her death and was trying to make her passing at least meaningful and comfortable.

On Sunday, March 2, 1997, John and Diana held what John believed to be their last conversation. John's impression was that Diana did not think she was going to die. John sat next to the hospital bed and stroked her arm. I sat across from them on the single bed for a few moments, but when I realized what he was doing, I left to go downstairs to the kitchen. I turned down the monitor and cried and cried and cried. From what I could tell, neither of them talked about death. Later that afternoon when Marisa drove John to the airport, John cried the whole way, and they had to stop in Gainsville, halfway to the airport, to get tissues.

On March 3rd, Dr. Maybach visited and recommended that we exercise her left arm to keep it from locking up. In her downturn, she was becoming immobile.

On March 4th, I wrote in my journal: "Last night/early this morning, Diana asked me what had made me stop laughing. She meant in our relationship. I told her that it was my selfishness, greed, and pettiness. Actually it was because of my anger—I didn't grow up in time to appreciate her. But she didn't either. This has been a blessed time for both of us. I think I am learning to stay in the present. The present is bearable and actually quite pleasant." Living in the present was part of my Zen practice, but I had strong leanings to living in the past and future. Taking care of Diana was forcing me to pay attention to the present.

Later in that journal entry, I listed my thoughts about what to place on her tombstone, and wrote the line, "Here lies a courageous mother who improved the direction of two families through her learning, love, and wisdom. She believed in us."

On March 11th, I gave her a toothbrush and then turned away to put some bowls on her tray. When I turned back, she was looking at the blankets, the toothbrush hanging from her mouth, spit draining from her lips. I removed the toothbrush and wiped her mouth.

A minute later, I gave her water by placing a straw in her mouth, and she sipped in, but didn't know to stop. Before I could put the basin beside her lips, she spit onto the pillow, thinking the basin was there. When she realized that the pillow was wet, she said, "A little trouble with eye-hand coordination."

On March 12th, her headaches had become so severe that we began Tylenol with Codeine. On March 16th, she was so congested from allergies that we began Claritan. By now she was taking six different drugs plus an array of vitamins.

On March 14th I wrote in my journal, "Diana is no longer the head of the family, so I have to take over. There is nothing wrong with being #1 in a family. I've never acted that way, but I can and do now." Diana was the first child in her family, and I was the third in mine. Over the years, I had deferred to her because she was so bright, because she had a larger vision, and also to repeat my own childhood position. We shared decision making in the most important issues—education of the children, childrearing, politics, religion, and finances. With her no longer able to function responsibly, I found myself making decisions that affected both of us, sometimes without conferring with her. This was new and strange for me.

Diana continued to weaken. I had to place my ear next to her mouth to hear her. I wrote in my journal on March 17th, "As the time draws near, I am sad. The time is near when she will leave us, and no amount of wishing or remembering will bring her back." The following day, I wrote, "I actually thought Diana would not make it to today. There are days when she is so weak." Also on the 18th I wrote to Maureen, "Yes, I have a sense these are extraordinary days—but they are so because everything is so downright ordinary—feeding, changing diapers, etc. The only time I have difficulty is when I'm not in the present." Paying attention to the motions of my hands and focusing on her body as I bathed her was very satisfying.

As I mentioned earlier, I think the cancer and her impending death forced us to drop our habits of anger and withdrawal, and to open up to each other. Once we did, our love for each other was there. This is something I have experienced many times since—that love underlies the turbulence of our lives. Love is not something we have to add; it is already here.

Also on March 18th I wrote, "Is it possible that she does not know she is dying? Is it possible she isn't? Is it possible she is in line for a recovery? Could she come back? Are we doing everything to make it possible for her to recover? If she were to have a recovery, would it come in the form of increased appetite, greater strength, clearer mind?" I then listed all the things we were doing for her. She had nutritious food, proper meds, and timely sponge baths, but not enough exercise; consequently, we moved her arms and legs because she had no strength to move them herself. Even though we did not know if she would recover, we had to act as if she would.

In early March, Brendan and Tracy announced that they were expecting a child to be born in early November. On Saturday, March 22nd, Marisa told Diana that she and Glen were expecting a child, also due in November. In the weeks that followed, Diana had moments of great sadness at the prospect of not being alive to hold them. I told her that she would be the grandmother of these children whether she was in this world or the spirit world, but I don't think these words was very comforting to her.

On March 28, Good Friday, I wrote in my journal, "Diana is particularly weak today—no breakfast, gurgling in her throat, and unable to talk more than a few phrases." I spent much of the day holding her hand; and twice, at 7:30 in the morning and again at 1:30 in the afternoon, I expected her to die. I certainly didn't expect her to make it through the weekend. We were no longer feeding her. Again, I wrote, "She knows she won't be around to be a physical grandmother. I told her she'll be a spiritual grandmother. I hope I'm doing the right thing by emphasizing the spiritual side of things."

March 29, Holy Saturday. "She has stopped eating. She breathes without gurgling, for the most part. We have her high up on her side. Last night, we had a long talk about going to the spirit world. She had questions, but she wasn't afraid. It was a good talk. I told her everything I knew." I expected her to die.

March 30, Easter. "She wakes at 4:30 p.m. and talks lucidly for half-an-hour about Brendan, and wants him to know she loves him. And then her talk becomes confused." The fact that it was Easter was not lost on me. I wondered if she, too, would experience a resurrection. Could she be a saint in the making? Could she, through her suffering, become holy enough to return in spirit form to heal other cancer patients?

March 31st, Diana slept most of the day. In the evening, Dr. Maybach visited with information on gene therapy. He said that none of the experimental gene treatments had been successful, but there was ongoing research. As I mentioned earlier, I, too, had checked out the possibility of Diana receiving gene therapy (having a tumor suppressor gene inserted in her brain), but a surgeon in Philadelphia said she would need to be strong enough to travel to the hospital and undergo two surgeries; at that point we couldn't slide her bed three feet to look out the window without her seizing. From my description of her progress after radiation, the surgeon guessed that her tumor had started growing immediately after treatment and her deterioration was a result of it invading the brain. He also said glioblastoma multiforme was the number one bad kind of cancer and that the average survival rate after diagnosis was nine months. I told him I would be surprised if she made it. Dr. Maybach said he would keep us informed about gene therapy should Diana gain enough strength to become eligible for treatment.

That night she was up from 9 to 12, frantic and agitated. I managed to forestall several seizures by keeping her calm.

On April 1st, Diana was again weak and slept most of the night and day. One of the nurses from Hospice thought her body might have been looking for ways to shut down.

On April 3rd, Diana asked me what would happen to her if she didn't get better. She had been practicing unbuttoning her pajama top "to keep up her dexterity," as she put it. I found it so sad when I saw her worrying about what might happen to her. I reassured her that people would be there to take care of her, but a part of her didn't believe me—and I never knew when that part would emerge.

The weather during the spring was beautiful—bright, clear, sunny days with flowers and trees in full bloom. We told her the weather was beautiful, but in early April, such a statement didn't mean much to her. She seized whenever we disturbed her—sometimes even when we changed the sheets and rolled her from side to side—no matter how slowly or gently.

I wrote to Maureen on April 8th, "I hug and kiss her with the same love and enthusiasm I did before we were married. She smells so sweet, and it feels so good to rub my cheek against her face. She is a joy to be around." The sweet smell of her skin came from the fruit we were feeding her, and, I would like to think, from the purity of her being.

By the middle of April, Diana was able to listen to the radio and comment on the programs, but the frantic pace of television sent her into seizure. On April 11th, I was sitting in the kitchen with Brendan and Tracy, while Marisa was eating dinner with Diana. Suddenly Marisa called me over the monitor, "Donald—Help." I ran upstairs to find Diana crying. I hugged her and asked her what was the matter. "I miss you, and I'm afraid of being alone," she said. This was the first time Diana had expressed fear of being alone.

On the 16th, her friends Sandy and Bruce visited for about 15–20 minutes. Then her left hand began to shake, and I asked her if she wanted to take a rest. She nodded. Also on the 16th, I was able to roll the hospital bed to the window without her seizing, and she looked out for the first time in months. Our neighbors across the street, Kay Oldaker and her son Harrison, were on the sidewalk, about 75 feet away. When I told Diana that Kay and Harrison were there, she said, "Hi." Her voice was weak, but her spirit was generous. Kay could not hear her, so I relayed Diana's greeting.

On the 17th, she was active, pulling the blanket off herself and pulling the pillow from under her head. With the bed still in front of the window, she pulled back the tabs on her diaper and pulled down one side. I jumped up and stopped her.

On Sunday morning, April 20th, I asked Diana about what she did on Sundays at home. I wanted to give her a chance to use her long-term memory because, during this period, her short-term memory was so unreliable. She spoke of several things that made me aware of the rich connections to her family. It felt so good to ask her questions she could answer. When I went downstairs to make breakfast, I heard, "Donald," on the monitor.

When I got back up, she said, "What were your Sundays like?" I found this to be so sweet, so generous of her.

When I thought of her childhood in Queens and Brooklyn, I felt sad because I never really got to know this part of her life. We never talked much about it, and I never appreciated how important friends and relatives were to her until she became sick.

Before we went to sleep that night, we talked about this being the best part of our marriage. We were closer than we had ever been, and there was genuine love for each other. "I think of you all the time," I told her.

"I do, too," she said.

On April 22nd, we were talking about our parents, and this is one of the few dialogues I copied down in my journal:

"I don't think my parents paid enough attention to me," she said.

"What did they not do that you wanted them to do?"

"Go to my basketball games. I wanted my father to go to my basketball games."

"Where was he?"

"Coming home from work."

"If your father were here, what would you say to him?"

She paused. "That I miss him."

I found it amazing that there was no blaming, no anger, no sorrow. Only love.

On April 23rd, we talked until late in the evening and I felt a little guilty that I had worn her out. When I turned her at 2:00 in the morning, she talked on and off until 5:00.

During this period, Diana's sleeping was erratic. Some days, she would be up for 24 hours at a stretch, while on other days she would take long naps in the morning and afternoon. At the time I thought she might be trying to stay awake to ward off death. In retrospect, I think her erratic sleeping was an early sign of recovery.

Hospice

The call to Hospice Support of Fauquier County was the most difficult call I made in the year and a half of Diana's illness. It was an admission of the seriousness of her illness. It also meant that I had been unable to take care of her by myself, and that her condition now required additional help. During her week in the hospital, I had come to accept the fact of her dying from this illness, but I still had to cope with the day-to-day consequences—one being that our home would now be open to people who would come to take care of her. Our home had always been private—open only to family, relatives, and close friends. Except for the rescue squad coming in January, the public stopped at the door.

The mental picture I had of hospice was of a somewhat run-down white stucco building with a sign out front at the end of Culpepper Street in Warrenton. Even though I had never been inside, I imagined barren rooms, whitewashed walls, a single bed with an ill person lying unconscious, a chair with the hospice person quietly reading a book, and light from a single pole lamp. My mental picture had no warmth in it. It was cold vigil.

I called hospice soon after Diana returned from the hospital. Dick Guizar, the director, answered the phone. I told him how difficult this call was. He said he understood, and the tone of his deep voice was reassuring. He took down my name, address, phone number, Diana's diagnosis and prognosis, and the name of her doctor. He said he would be by the house in a few hours to do an assessment.

I remember having mixed feelings about telling Dick about Diana's prognosis. I needed the help hospice offered, and I thought they provided assistance only for the last month of a person's life. I told Dick that Dr. Maybach didn't expect her to live past Christmas, eleven months away, but I also told him she might go in a month. I knew it was possible, but I didn't want to believe it. I didn't like thinking about her dying so soon and really didn't think she was that sick. I was hoping the surgery, radiation, and two treatments of chemo had done the trick.

At this point, I also did not respect the accuracy of the medical profession's prognosis because I was focusing on the few exceptions I had heard about. I wanted Diana to be an exception. So a part of me thought I was lying to Dick about how long she would live.

Dick's visit was warm and friendly. We sat at the kitchen table for about fifteen minutes during which he asked me questions to fill out his assessment form—questions about Diana's medications and treatments, her ability to get about, the care she needed for bathing, how much we knew about the illness, and the kind of help I needed. I told him I could use someone for about two hours each on Monday, Wednesday, and Friday, preferably around lunch time so that someone could be with Diana when I prepared lunch, ran out to the store for food and medicine, or made calls to doctors, pharmacists, and health insurance people. We settled on hospice workers coming from 11:00 a.m. to 1:00 p.m. each of those three days. I also needed to borrow a wheel chair, a bedside commode, and a bath chair. At the time, they had over 40 hospital beds, but all were on loan.

I recall his meeting Diana as being similar to my meeting a new neighbor—small talk and a few questions. What made it unusual was that it occurred in a bedroom, and Diana was in one of the two single beds. I think she was pleased that I was getting help to take care of her. She knew I had a long history of self-reliance (a fancy name for being shy about asking for help), and I think she understood how desperate I must have been to call in hospice. In addition, this was the first visit by someone other than family and friends. Our home was now open to strangers.

As it turned out, the hospice office had moved from Culpepper Street to North Fifth Street, two blocks from our home. It contained a reception area, a meeting room in the back, two offices, and a storage area for equipment and supplies. Their equipment included hospital beds when available, bedside commodes, wheel chairs, wound supplies, IV stands, bandages, and the like. It also included cases of Ensure, chucks, and disposable diapers.

One of the most valuable services provided by hospice was a group of people I could talk to about Diana's condition. When volunteers came to the house, I briefed them on Diana's condition before they sat with her. Such briefings were very helpful to me because it forced me to evaluate her condition daily. Some of the volunteers were nurses, in particular, Mittie Wallace, who came twice a week for the entire year. Mittie and I talked about Diana's medications, ways to bathe and change her diaper, ways to prevent bedsores, exercises to keep her from becoming stiff, and food that was good for her to eat.

Dick Guizar's term of office came to a close soon after we began working with hospice, and Joy LaBarron became the new director. Joy was a cheery, warm, and compassionate person, and my calls to her over the year made a huge difference. At the time, her brother was a pharmacist in medical school, studying to become a doctor, and from Joy and her brother I got valuable information on medications. I talked to our son, John, daily about Diana's meds, and with the additional information from Joy, I was able to have intelligent conversations with Dr. Maybach. Joy also gave me comfort and encouragement, and from time to time reminded me to take care of myself. I knew if I didn't, Diana might end up in a hospital or nursing home, and I did not want that.

After Diana died, I learned from Joy and Mittie that some people don't know how to talk about terminal illnesses and death. In fact, some spouses don't even talk to the patient about the illness. Joy told me that some people had come to the hospice office and burst out crying because they knew they could finally talk to someone about caring for a loved one with a terminal illness. My talks with Joy over the phone and with the hospice volunteers who came to our home were easy for me because they understood what I was talking about. I didn't have to explain basic thoughts and emotions; they asked intelligent questions and offered helpful advice.

Joy also said that some doctors were reluctant to refer patients to hospice, and, in fact, referred them only weeks or days before they were about to die. These doctors saw such referrals as a sign of their giving up on the patient. I think we were very fortunate because Dr. Maybach immediately saw the larger picture and, without ever giving up the search for a cure, humbly referred me to home health care and hospice. By the way, Hospice Support of Fauquier County is a support hospice as opposed to a medical hospice. A support hospice is run by volunteers, and it does not accept Medicare funding or payment from insurance companies. As with other volunteer organizations, only a few positions are salaried, and as with all incorporated organizations, they have bylaws and a board of directors. I had heard that you had to be in the last month of your life for hospice to help you, but that was not true. You merely have to be terminally ill. A support hospice also accepts patients who are getting radiation or chemotherapy, patients technically considered curable.

Hospice never makes first contact—the patient or family must do that. At the time, our hospice has an average caseload of about 16 patients at a time, with a high of 22 and a low of 10. It maintained strict confidentiality: files were locked and available only to the directors. Diana's name was never used when volunteers talked to spouses or friends—she was merely a patient on High Street.

As director, one of Joy's jobs was to match the volunteers to the patient. Some volunteers prefer to help the patient with such things as feeding and bathing, while others prefer to talk or read quietly. Because Diana was bedridden and needed considerable help, Joy selected volunteers who could feed, bathe, and change her. For medical reasons, their only limitation was feeding her medications. They could place her meds on the bedside table when Diana was able to take them herself, but they could not administer them to her.

In the early 1800's, the term "hospice" referred to a house where travelers could rest or where the destitute or sick could be cared for. Such houses were usually owned by a religious order.

The modern hospice movement was started by a British woman named Dr. Cicely Saunders who founded St. Christopher's in London in 1967, an inpatient hospice. The first hospice in America, the Connecticut Hospice, Inc., was founded in Branford, Connecticut, in 1974. Between these two dates, Dr. Elizabeth Kubler Ross published *On Death and Dying* (1969) identifying the five stages through which many terminally ill patients progress. She based her book on interviews with over 500 dying patients, and argued both for home care and for patients having a choice in decisions that affect their lives. In 1972, testifying before a US Senate Special Committee on Aging, Dr. Kubler Ross said, "We live in a very peculiar death-denying society. We isolate both the dying and the old, and it serves a purpose. They are reminders of our own mortality. We should not institutionalize people. We can give families more help with home care and visiting nurses, giving the families and the patients the spiritual, emotional, and financial help in order to facilitate the final care at home." In 1977, there are over 2,400 hospices in the United States.

Nine hospice volunteers visited Diana over a period of 13 months: Mittie Wallace, Diane Harbaugh, Carolyn Strong, Fran Foster, Pat Gould, Kathy Fitz, Mary Katz, Susie Barber, and Betty Ruffner. Mittie, Diane, Carolyn, and Fran came regularly, with Mittie coming to see Diana twice a week for over a year, mostly on Monday and Wednesdays from 11:00 a.m. to1:00 p.m. I rarely stayed in the room while Mittie visited because, as I said earlier, I needed to get food and meds from the store, or talk to doctors, pharmacists, and insurance people on the phone.

Mittie brought laughter. Just as some people might punctuate their conversations with a look or a gesture, Mittie laughed. When I left the room, Diana would be in a good mood, and when I returned an hour-and-a-half later, she would be laughing. Diana's laugh was soft and gentle, and after she lost her eyesight, her laugh replaced the light in her eyes.

Mittie also brought girl talk, a kind of talk between women that is different from talk between women and men. Mittie and Diana talked about rearing children, handling parents, husbands, and relatives, and countless other topics. Because Mittie was also a nurse, she brought practical knowledge about how to keep Diana healthy. I recall in particular one conversation with Mittie about giving Diana fruit juices. I had been giving her fresh orange juice. When I mentioned to Mittie that one of our friends said that non-acidic fruit juices, such as mango juice, would be better for Diana so that her skin would not break down when she wet her diapers, Mittie said that Diana also needed the acidity in orange juice and that it would not cause a problem. Consequently, from time to time I squeezed oranges for Diana.

I had picked up the tricks of the trade on taking care of a bed-ridden patient during the week in the hospital, and Mittie helped me to develop these skills further—such as turning Diana every two hours, bathing her, dressing and undressing her, sanitary procedures when changing diapers, and the like. Typically, I served Diana breakfast, washed her face and hands, and, of course, changed her diaper, or helped her onto the bedside commode before Mittie arrived at 11:00 a.m. Mittie often gave her a sponge bath, a foot massage, and checked Diana's scalp, and sometimes she would help Diana complete a series of exercises to regain her strength.

Mittie thought there was an aura about Diana that made her the energy center of the room, and she admired Diana's peace, courage, and acceptance of her situation. She also saw Diana regularly giving a piece of herself to others, and noticed that even though the very bright intellectual side of Diana had come to grips with her having cancer, she still used synonyms to talk about dying.

In one of their conversations about children, Diana told Mittie, "You have to clear out the cobwebs in the mind if you're going to enjoy your children." In a conversation about Mittie's somewhat troubled relationship with her mother, Diana said, "You have to love your mother, or you'll be depriving your children of their grandmother." These comments show Diana's wisdom and her children-centered worldview. Mittie once asked Diana what was the one thing in life that she wanted, and Diana replied, "I want my children to be happy. There are no tradeoffs for happiness." I have often quoted this last sentence, and it serves as a guide for my actions.

Mittie had a gift for asking the large questions in a non-threatening way. She asked Diana what was the one thing she regretted, and Diana told her about having to fire an employee in his 30's who was diabetic. According to Diana, he didn't take care of himself, he didn't take his insulin, he drank, and he didn't eat right. He went into diabetic comas several times while at work, and paramedics were called in. Eventually he wasn't able to do his job. Diana kept him on for an additional six months, and they eventually came to an agreement that he had to leave. He moved to Florida, but had no one to take care of him. He died shortly after that. I can imagine Diana's condition making her even more aware of the terrible situation this employee was in when he had no one to take care of him and wasn't in the habit of taking care of himself.

Diana could be adamant. She wasn't going to let the cancer take over without a fight. But she also knew when the time was not right for her to exercise. One day, Mittie came in, and Diana told her she wasn't going to exercise that morning. Mittie tried to persuade her, but nothing changed her mind. I also saw this fierce determination when she told us she was getting out to shop for Christmas gifts for the grandchildren. We all knew from the way that she said it that there was no point in discussing it.

One day, while Mittie was visiting and I was preparing lunch in the kitchen, a young cardinal crashed into the windowpane in Diana's room. It lay on the porch roof, stunned and unmoving. Diana called over the baby monitor for me to come up and take care of the bird. I got a small cardboard box, opened the window, and put the bird in the box. Its heart was beating rapidly. I covered it and by the time I walked down the stairs and outside onto the front lawn, the bird had recovered and was strong enough to fly away. Mittie said Diana considered me her "knight in shining armor" for rescuing the bird.

Diana went through a period when she felt insecure about my going off to the store even though Mittie was staying with her. She would ask me yet another question or remind me of just one more thing as I was about to leave the room. Finally, Mittie had to reassure her, "He's just a phone call away," she said.

Mittie listened as Diana talked about my getting only one hour of sleep at night.

"I'm concerned about you, Don," Mittie said.

"I'm fine," I told her. "There are nights when I catch up." I knew that Diana was talking to Mittie in order to get me to take better care of myself. I reassured Diana that I was in good health.

About me, she once told Mittie, "I know he loves me." I felt so grateful that my reiteration of "I love you," had made it though.

Hallucinations

One day during the week Diana spent in the hospital, I came back from class, and Tracy said that Diana had seen a dog figurine that disappeared when she tried to touch it. The next day, I was in the room with her and saw her reach gently into the air as if she were trying to touch something with her long, beautiful fingers.

"Something there?" I asked, being a little unsure of how to handle this.

"A figurine," she said, looking at the point in front of her fingers.

"Can I help," I asked, not knowing what I would do if she said yes.

"No, it's OK," she said, then returned her hand to the bed. The hallucination must have subsided because her attention returned to the room.

In March 1997, a month after she returned home from the hospital, she would occasionally see cats, dogs, and other animals. She would ask us to take them from the room, which we did. We knew they weren't there, we knew they were hallucinations, but we pretended they were real because we didn't want to upset her or argue with her. We knew how easily she seized when she was upset, so we kept conflict and arguments to an absolute minimum. We pretended to scoop the critters up into our hands or catch them, then walk them out into the hall or downstairs and out of the house. Sometimes, the critters would be in the room; other times they would be on the bed. We would pretend to see them, move our hands to where she said they were, catch them, and take them away. Sometimes, we would move our hands to where they were on the bed and miss them—and she would tell us again to get the critter, and we had to try again. I don't understand how she could see the critters move in our hands if the reality of our hands had no physical contact with the hallucination in her mind.

Everyone who took care of her during this period knew to play along, to pretend that we could see the critters.

Hallucinations are, to the person hallucinating, real. This is the lesson I learned early on, and knowing this really helped me throughout the period Diana had them. Hallucinations have no basis in reality, but they are real sights, sounds, or smells triggered by synapse connections in the brain. We will never know if the cancer, the surgery, or the radiation caused them. For Diana, the hallucinations were sights as real as images we see with our eyes. In the beginning, we tried not to disagree with her because they were so real to her, and it was easy to remove them. As time went on, however, the critters became more frequent, and some days we spent hours taking them out of the room only for them to return minutes later. Some visitors remarked about how patient we were to take them out, hour after hour. We thought it best for her that we pretend to see them, too, and to remove them.

In April, Diana saw a horse. She never described it, but she loved seeing it, and from that I assumed it was beautiful. She would ask us to take the horse out of the room, so we pretended to lead it by a halter downstairs and out into the back yard. It returned, of course, so, in an attempt to make it more difficult to return, we told her we had taken it into the field behind our property. We were trying to use logic to forestall a hallucination.

At times, Diana would ask, "How is the horse?" Whoever was in the room would make up an answer, and, as we soon discovered, a different answer.

Tracy: "It's in the back yard, and it's fine."
Glen: "It's in the field eating hay."
Donald: "It's in the front yard eating grass."

We soon learned to confer and make our stories consistent. When the horse kept coming back, I thought we should tell her we had found a place for it to live.

There was a beautiful horse farm called Eastwood on Old Auburn Road, the road on the way to Brendan's house that was then owned by the Rogers family. We told Diana that we had talked to one of the Rogers who was willing to take the horse and pasture it for free, but that it would be several days before he could come and get the horse. I added this delay to allow her time to get used to the idea. As far as I could tell, she was no longer seeing the horse, but she was very concerned about it. On Saturday, we told her he had called and would be over on Sunday. On Sunday, we told her he had come to the back pasture, had led the horse into his trailer, and before leaving, assured us he would take good care of him. Diana asked about the horse from time to time, and we'd tell her that he was happy with the other horses on the Rogers farm.

Unfortunately, the hallucinations did not stop with the horse. Diana then saw snakes, lots of them, and some of them frightened her. I'm terrified of snakes, and if I had seen them, I would have screamed and broken out in a sweat. Diana was relatively calm, brushing them aside before asking us to remove them. A few times she would cower and look up, so I think some of them were cobras or snakes that reared up. Mittie was very calm talking to Diana about the snakes, and even took one of them for her daughter to use in a school science project. The rest of us just got rid of them.

At first I would say, "No, there aren't any snakes here," because I didn't want her to be alarmed, but instead she felt discounted. I was quite willing to remove them each time she saw them, but their appearances became so frequent that they were interrupting my feeding her, my bathing her, and our listening to the radio. I wanted to find a way to let her know that I thought they were imaginary even though she saw them as real.

"I'm having a hard time taking care of you with all these snakes," I said. "I can't see them, and I'm not sure they're real."

I was looking for a way to talk about them without dismissing what she saw. She didn't reply, but I could tell she was thinking it over. After a few days, she said, "Whenever you don't see the snakes, say, 'This seems a little odd. I think we should check it out.' That will be our little code."

"Brilliant," I said. It thought it was a wonderful way to handle the hallucinations. I wrote these two sentences on a yellow post-it note, memorized it, and asked everyone to use these sentences whenever she had hallucinations.

It worked. Thereafter, she accepted our telling her that we thought her hallucinations weren't real.

After the horse and the snakes, Diana saw a pond behind our house. I was grateful that this hallucination was not something that could come into the room, so I never dissuaded her from believing in it.

Late in April, Diana saw a kitten next to her and became alarmed that I might harm him as I leaned on the bed. "Watch out for the kitty," she said. "Do you think you could get a box for him? I went downstairs, got a cardboard box from the kitchen, placed the kitty in it, and took the box into the hall. When I returned, there was a second kitten in the room that I then dispatched in the same manner. "What did you do with them," she asked.

"I put them in Marisa's round cat bed—the one her cats didn't like, remember? And I put the cat bed in the master bedroom."

"That's good. They'll be out of the way there," she said. Later that day, she saw a third kitten which I placed with the others. She seemed pleased that I was taking such good care of them.

The next morning, she said, "I'd like to see the kittens."

"*Oh, shit*," I thought. "OK. Let me get them," I said, and walked into the master bedroom, thinking fast about what to tell her. I remembered the early years of our marriage when we had raised Siamese kittens to help pay for grad school. At one time, we had 13 cats in the house. One of the mother cats that Diana named Tup Tim after the girl in "*The King and I*" was pregnant and due to deliver at the same time Diana was due with Marisa. The cat waited until Diana returned from the hospital, then gave birth in the kitchen and carried the kittens one by one up to our bed in the master bedroom where Diana was sleeping.

I decided to use that experience as an excuse for not being able to bring her the kittens. I walked out of the master bedroom and down the hall, looking into the other two bedrooms, then yelled back to Diana. "She must have moved them. I can't find them, and I don't know where they are." I continued to look throughout the house, calling back, "I can't find them." When I returned to the bedroom, I looked at Diana. Her face looked calm, and she seemed content with my explanation. The cat hallucinations subsided after that.

Around seven o'clock on most evenings, a car would race up the street with its boom box blaring. Diana was convinced that this car, which was real, was driven by hoodlums who one day would hit someone. She often asked me to call the police. Finally I gave in and went downstairs, and pretended to call. It was an odd coincidence that the car did not appear for several days. When it returned, Diana said, "There they go again," in a disparaging tone of voice.

One Saturday night, she heard something in the house and quickly became convinced it was an intruder. "Call the police, call the police," she insisted.

"I think it's just a noise. I don't think anyone is in the house, but I'll check." I walked from room to room, upstairs and down, pretending to search the house. "I don't see anyone," I said.

She seemed satisfied, but minutes later she heard another noise. "You have to call the police," she said, quite agitated.

"OK. I'll call them from downstairs," I said. I thought it would do no harm, so I went downstairs and pretended to call 911. I returned to the bedroom to wait with her, and, after ten minutes, said. "The police are here. I'm going downstairs to talk with them." When I returned, I told her the police agreed to search the house. I waited for a short while, again went downstairs, and returned to say, "They haven't found anything, and they think we're safe here."

Diana wasn't satisfied. "I'm sure someone's in the house." She soon heard another noise, and again insisted that I call 911. Again, I pretended that the police had come, and this time I said, "The police did find someone and took him away." Instead of making her feel more secure, it made her more alarmed. I knew I had made a mistake, but I didn't know how to get out of this ever expanding story.

"What did he look like? What was he doing? Where did they find him? Is he going to stay in jail?" If it had not been so upsetting for Diana, it would have been a great way to spend a Saturday evening. She didn't settle down until after midnight.

The next morning, she wanted to know what the police were doing with the intruder. I decided to downplay the arrest by giving her as little information as possible. During the week, she asked me, "What did the papers say?"

"I don't know. The paper comes on Wednesday. I'll let you know."

Come Wednesday, she asked me, "Could you read me the paper about the intruder?"

"Yes, there's an account of him in the police section, but I'm busy now. Can I read it to you later?" I was planning to paraphrase an already existing account of an arrest. When Tracy arrived on Saturday, she actually did walk off with the page I needed. When she returned it, Marisa, quite by mistake, took it home with her; and this went on for weeks. Eventually, Diana stopped asking. But I learned my lesson. After that, I tried to avoid making up stories.

As I mentioned earlier, in the middle of March 1997, Tracy announced that she and Brendan were expecting. A week later, Marisa sat across the bed watching Diana as she slept and whispered to me, "You'll never guess what!"

"You're pregnant," I said, joking.

"Yes," she said. I was surprised and delighted.

Several weeks after these announcements, Diana began seeing babies in the house. The first baby she saw she named Jo, and a few weeks later a second baby arrived who she named Caroline. After a while I realized, and so did Diana, that these were the names of our married children's mother-in-laws, Jo Faunce and Carolyn Chidester. Diana was pleased with the coincidence.

By the end of April Diana was preoccupied with these imaginary babies and spent her waking hours taking care of them. Of course, because she was bedridden, she gave me very specific instructions about what to do. Jo, being the older, was "into everything" as the expression goes, including playing with kitchen knives.

A year before Diana became ill, she watched Matthew Margolis train dogs on a National Public Television fundraiser, and subsequently ordered the tape in which Margolis used a high pitched "Woof!" voice to praise the dogs and a low-pitched voice to correct them. When Jo brandished a knife, Diana would say in a very low voice, "No, Jo, give Daddy the knife," then praised her in a high-toned voice, "Good girl. That's a good girl, Jo."

One day, Diana was very alarmed. "What's the matter," I asked.

"There are two boys standing on the roof dropping clay flower pots on Jo's head."

"Oh no, I'll stop them," which I pretended to do.

"You have to take her to the emergency room. She'll need stitches." So I pretended to do that, too.

By now, the hallucinations of Jo and Caroline were robbing us of our relationship with each other. Taking care of Diana was easy when she appreciated what I did for her, but when the appreciation evaporated, I felt exhausted. In addition, these hallucinations had become a problem for Diana because Jo and Carolyn were constantly getting into danger, and she was spending all her energy taking care of them.

I talked to John about the hallucinations, and he recommended the drug Risperdal. I called Dr. Maybach who prescribed it on May 27, 1997. That night her speech was slow and she was groggy. The next day she was a little calmer, but she did see an alligator and had me call 911. I reported to her that the game warden had come by and carted off the reptile. She was groggy the rest of the week, and even though she continued to have hallucinations, she was calmer.

Risperdal usually takes effect in two weeks, and about this time she asked to be taken off the drug because it made her groggy, so we took her off. The hallucinations continued, but were mild until the 16th of June when I asked her if she would like to go back on Risperdal to control the hallucinations. She agreed, so we continued with a very low dosage. On June 19th, Diana wanted to talk about the things we should do differently in rearing the babies she was seeing. She thought we should do the following:

- listen to "Woof!"
- refrain from saying "no" with their names because it is demoralizing;
- read books for successful strategies for rearing children;
- and get them involved with sports, theater, and the arts.

As the Risperdal decreased the hallucinations, Diana noticed that the babies did not talk. "Do you think there is something wrong with them?" she asked.

"Thomas Aquinas didn't talk until he was five years old," I told her, and Einstein didn't talk until he was much older."

This mollified her for a while, but then she noticed that Jo and Caroline weren't gaining weight. One morning when Mittie was scheduled to visit from Hospice, Diana said, "Could you bring Jo to me so she can nurse?"

When Mittie walked in, Diana had her pajama top unbuttoned and her breasts exposed, cradling Jo in her arms, trying to nurse her. When Jo didn't nurse, she had me take her back to the crib in the master bedroom.

We had been talking about hallucinations, and I was hoping that Diana would draw the conclusion by herself that Jo and Caroline were not real. As she became more concerned with their not growing and their possibly having birth defects, I knew I would have to ease her into talking about them as hallucinations. On Thursday evening, June 26th, I sat on the chair next to the bed, and as gently as I could, I said, "I think there might be a connection between the babies being quiet, their not growing, your taking Risperdal, and your having fewer hallucinations." I was very careful not to draw the conclusion for her.

After a few moments, she said, "You mean the babies might not be real?" then burst out crying—sobbing as a mother sobs at the death of a child. I cried with her because she was heartbroken. I also cried because she might have felt humiliated knowing that others knew they were hallucinations when she didn't.

The next day, when her friends Sandy and Bruce visited, she told them about the babies and again cried. We mourned their loss for about a week, crying over and over. She so loved those babies.

Diana took Risperdal the rest of her life to control hallucinations. If the hallucinations increased, I increased the Risperdal—always telling John what I was doing, making sure I was within the guidelines established by Dr. Maybach. The dosage never rose above 1 milligram a day and eventually dropped to a maintenance dosage of half that. The hallucinations continued, but Diana did not seem disturbed by them. I believe that she came to recognize certain "sights" as unreal. I think she saw the babies again but never allowed herself to believe they were real. We knew she was seeing something when she swept her hand across in front of her, and I think she knew she was having an hallucination when we would hesitate immediately after she told us she saw something.

At one point in the summer of 1997, Diana said to Mittie, "I want you to be honest. Do you see the snakes?"

"No," Mittie said.

"Is there a pond behind the house?" Diana asked.

"No, I don't see one."

"And Donald didn't speak to you first?"

Mittie laughed and said, "No, Donald didn't speak to me first."

I think this brief conversation with Mittie greatly helped her to understand the hallucinations.

Meds

For 56 years, we were healthy. From time to time Diana took Claritin for allergies, or one of us in the family took an antibiotic for an infection, but otherwise we didn't take prescription drugs and rarely took over-the-counter drugs.

I think Diana's undergraduate degree in chemistry played a role in her understanding of drugs, and her acceptance of them as helpful and necessary made it easier for me to give them to her. I, on the other hand, saw them as a symbol of our failure to remain healthy, and throughout her illness looked for ways to lower her dosages or eliminate a medication altogether. Only when John reminded me of the consequences of not giving them to her did I see them as an aide to her well-being.

Meds Log

John must have known how important and difficult it would be to keep track of meds because as soon as we returned to Fairfax from Boston, he bought a daily calendar, one for teachers because it was October and the only ones available were for the academic year that starts in August. For the first week after Diana returned home from surgery, he listed each day's meds:

A.M.	Zantac150 (1 pill)
	Dilantin 100 mg (1 pill)
	Decadron 2 mg (2 pills)
Lunch	Dilantin 100 mg (1 pill)
	Decadron 2 mg (2 pills)
Dinner	Dilantin 100 mg (1 pill)
	Decadron 2 mg (2 pills)
Hs	Zantac 150 mg (1 pill)
	Dilantin 100 mg (1 pill)
	Decadron 2 mg (2 pills)

"Hs" (hour of sleep) meds were taken at bedtime. Each time I gave Diana meds, I crossed them off with a yellow high–lighter. In February, 1997, we were given a pill organizer in which I placed the pills once a week, then entered the time, the drug, and the dosage in the meds log each time I gave them to her. I also used the log to keep track of doctor appointments, treatments, physical therapy sessions, and observations on her health (e.g., "wakes with headache").

The meds log saved us numerous times, mostly when I was so tired I had trouble remembering which drug I had just given her. I am so grateful that there were only a few instances when I was unable to keep track of them.

Taking Meds

In the beginning, Diana took her own medications. As she progressed through radiation, she became weak and could not remember to take them, or remember the correct dosage. Eventually, I took the pills out of the bottles and placed them in a saucer for her.

When she became weak, she could no longer swallow the pills on her own, and we would find a dry pill lodged between her lip and her gum hours after she had taken it. We then resorted to crushing the pills, at first between two spoons, then later in a mortar and pestle, before mixing the powder in applesauce. Capsules, of course, we broke apart with our fingers and dropped the meds directly into the applesauce. Because the pills were bitter, the applesauce had to be very sweet. During the time that our sister-in-law, Martha Batch, stayed with us, she made a delectable applesauce from fresh apples, butter, cinnamon, and sugar, which Diana loved. Later, when Martha returned home, we used applesauce from the store and added sugar if necessary.

From the beginning, I had trouble splitting pills. When I cut them with a sharp paring knife on a cutting board, I often fragmented them. I will always be grateful to Dr. Maybach for showing me how to hold them firmly in my fingers, and snap them in half along the scored line. With practice, it became easy.

As I mention elsewhere, Diana took meds slowly and carefully, never rushing, never gulping the liquid she used to wash them down, never gagging on them. Watching her take meds was for me akin to watching the Japanese Tea Ceremony—a ritual filled with attention. It calmed me, made me slow down, and brought my focus to my hands and fingers.

By the way, our Hospice volunteers were not allowed to administer meds. I believe they were allowed to place them on the table so Diana could take them herself, but they could not give them to her directly. It may be different in different parts of the country, but this was our situation here.

A Misunderstanding

In January, 1997, Dr. Susan Lord suggested that Diana take a few drops of Rescue Remedy, a calming agent made from five flowers: Star-of-Bethlehem; Rock Rose; Impatiens; Cherry Plum; and Clematis. Rescue Remedy is one of 38 flower and herbal remedies developed by Dr. Edward Bach, a British bacteriologist who studied the connection between negative states of mind and physical illness. The theory behind Rescue Remedy is that if a person's energy system is restored to normal after a traumatic event, such as discovering one has brain cancer and has undergone surgery and radiation, that it will be easier for the person to heal.

I don't know how I got Dr. Lord's instructions confused, but I did. I thought Rescue Remedy was an alternative anti–nausea medication, that is a substitute for Zofran. Diana had a few instances of nausea in January, especially following the second chemotherapy treatment, so I gave her Rescue Remedy each time she felt nauseous, six drops under her tongue, thinking that its side effects would be less debilitating than the ones mentioned above for Zofran. Rescue Remedy did not curb the nausea, and after a few weeks, I switched to Zofran that worked beautifully, and completely without side effects. When I told Dr. Lord that Rescue Remedy didn't control the nausea, she was surprised that I was using it for that purpose. I was so embarrassed that I had made this mistake, and I felt responsible for causing Diana to suffer needlessly.

Looking back, there was probably no way to avoid some mistakes like this. I know now that I am a visual learner and that I find it difficult to remember verbal instructions or directions. It is as if I have to translate the words into images in order to follow and remember them. I also know that Diana's whole system was rebelling at this time from the radiation and chemotherapy, and that no medication was going to reverse the damage done by these treatments. And I wish I had had Mechthild Scheffer's book, *Bach Flower Therapy*, because I could have looked it up and avoided all the confusion.

Drug Information Profile

In January of 1997, I knew Diana's weakness was coming from the radiation and chemotherapy treatments, but I also suspected that the meds were also contributing to her downturn. Fueling my suspicion was the one-page Drug Information Profile that accompanied each prescription, and included the name of the drug, its common uses, how to use the medication, various cautions, and finally its possible side effects. She was taking Zofran to prevent nausea and vomiting, and the possible side effects statement read as follows: "Side effects that may go away during treatment, include headache, constipation, stomach pain, weakness, and dry mouth. If they continue or are bothersome, check with your doctor. If you notice other effects not listed above, contact your doctor, nurse, or pharmacist."

She was also taking Dexamethasone to prevent swelling in the brain, and the possible side effects statement for this was:

> "SIDE EFFECTS that may go away during treatment include difficulty sleeping, mood changes, nervousness, increased appetite, or indigestion. If they continue or are bothersome, check with your doctor. CHECK WITH YOUR DOCTOR AS SOON AS POSSIBLE if you experience swelling of feet or legs; unusual weight gain; black tarry stools; vomiting material that looks like coffee grounds; severe nausea or vomiting; changes in menstrual periods; headache; muscle weakness; or prolonged sore throat, cold or fever. If you notice other effects not listed above, contact your doctor, nurse, or pharmacist."

I found this statement alarming, and often when we talked to our doctors about meds, I asked if we could lower the dosage. In February, 1997, when I told Dr. Maybach how I felt about the possible side effects listed on the Drug Information Profile, he explained that drug companies had to list them for legal purposes, but for most people, the side effects were minimal or non-existent. This put my mind at ease.

I still had to remind myself of what John had told me previously, that any side effects of the drugs were less severe than the consequences of not taking them. As it turned out, the only side effects I noticed were sleepiness from Risperdal and constipation from Codeine.

Donald Gallehr

Triangulation of Data on Meds

The teacher-research field developed by my colleague Marian Mohr and others referred to checking three different sources against each other as a triangulation of data. When researching drugs, I triangulated the data by gathering information from three sources: printed material, our local pharmacists, and our son John, a doctor trained in the application of these drugs. Then I conferred with Dr. Eric Maybach, our family physician. The printed sources I used were *The Mayo Clinic Family Health Book*, and the book *Worst Pills, Best Pills II* published in 1993 by the Public Citizen's Health Research Group founded by Ralph Nader, written to help prevent patients, especially older patients, from receiving drugs that are harmful.

I want to digress for a moment in order to make a point about drugs. I recently had a mild cold which within a week turned into a sinus infection. Rather than wait it out, rather than drown it with orange juice, vitamins, and home-made chicken soup, I took an over-the-counter decongestant. The label cautioned users not to use it if they have high blood pressure or any one of several other conditions. I have borderline hypertension but thought that its being an over-the-counter drug made it safe.

The drug did a beautiful job of drying up my sinuses, but it also gave me the first anxiety attack of my life, and when I attempted to donate blood, I was refused because my blood pressure had risen from 128/78 to 160/106.

I relate this story because it is this experience and others like it over the years that have made me very cautious about taking both over-the-counter and prescription drugs.

In one instance, this caution and my using a triangulation of data, stopped me from giving Diana a drug called Darvocet. I believe it was prescribed early on in Diana's illness for severe pain, and we filled the prescription, but we never had occasion to use it. In the second week of March 1997, she began to have headaches. When I looked in *Worst Pills, Best Pills II*, I found they recommended against taking it: "We recommend that you do not use it [Darvocet] because it is no more effective than aspirin or codeine and it is much more dangerous than aspirin." It went on to say, "Most studies show that propoxyphene is less effective than aspirin and that it has a potential for addiction and overdose." (Wolfe et al. 1993, p. 279)

When I spoke to the pharmacist, he said that some people do have an adverse reaction to Darvocet, but there is no way to know before trying it.

John's opinion was that it was a much more powerful drug, and because it was an opiate designed to block pain, it could become addictive.

The consequence of my doing my homework was that when I talked to Dr. Maybach, I understood him when he said that we could use either Tylenol with Codeine or Darvocet, but we were to limit the Darvocet to three times a day. I chose to give her Tylenol with Codeine that I thought would be more effective and less dangerous. If Tylenol with Codeine did not work, then I would call Dr. Maybach and tell him I wanted to switch to Darvocet. Fortunately, Tylenol with Codeine worked.

Calling in Meds and Picking Them Up

Anyone who is on meds on a regular basis knows how important it is that the doctor or someone in his office call in the prescription when you request it. In the beginning, I would call the doctor's office on the day the prescription ran out, and assume it would be called in immediately. I would then run to the drug store only to discover that it had not been called in. I would either wait while the pharmacist called the doctor's office, or return the next day. Because I had only a short period when someone would be in the house with Diana, time was crucial.

I eventually became good at calling in refill requests when the prescription was sufficiently used up so that the insurance company would honor it, and also in time to pick it up before we had run out. There were instances of the wrong data being entered into the computer by the pharmacist, but these were rare. There was also one instance when Dr. Maybach was at a conference when we needed a prescription of Claritin. Fortunately, his wife was able to contact another doctor who handled it.

Who Is In Charge?

One of the problems we encountered in the first three months of Diana's illness was that she had three doctors—a surgeon, an oncologist, and a radiation oncologist. While each one asked how Diana was doing, it seemed like no one was in charge of the overall picture. When Diana spent a week in the hospital late in January 1997, Dr. Maybach became our primary physician, and he monitored her medications. Nevertheless, even with daily contact with John, and with telephone access to Dr. Maybach, we still had a few problems. One was with the drug Tegretol that Dr. Azzam prescribed November 27, 1996, to control facial seizures. The following February, Dr. Moore prescribed Neurontin also to control seizures. So, by February, Diana was taking Dilantin, Tegretol, and Neurontin, each to control seizures. I eventually asked our pharmacist about the overlapping nature of these drugs, and he agreed that we didn't need all three. Consequently, when her seizures subsided in May, I tapered the Tegretol. When Dr. Maybach returned from vacation and visited the house, I told him what I had done. He said he had no problem with my decision.

The point I want to make here is that even though we had an excellent system of administering meds, I was the only one who was in a position to keep tabs on all parts of it, and I had very limited knowledge of this field. Because I was the only one who saw the subtle changes in her condition each day, every day, doctors had to rely on the accuracy of my observations and reports. There were times when I wanted to feel the effects of the drugs myself, but, considering the kinds of drugs (after all, this was not aspirin), this was impossible.

I have come to appreciate the importance of well-written nurse's notes and doctor's notes so that when the patient or the primary care giver is unable to maintain continuity, such information can bridge the gap. Looking back, I could have used a Meds 101 course at the beginning of Diana's illness. And I do have to admit that despite my reluctance to give her medications, Diana had a much more comfortable last year because of them.

Before finishing this chapter, I want to say that we were very fortunate with the pharmacists who helped us—the ones who not only fulfilled our prescriptions, but those who answered our questions. Several times our pharmacists managed to clear up confusion with the insurance companies, and those who came to know us went out of their way to ask how Diana was doing.

And one more thing: Diana never once complained about the taste of the drugs. Near the end of her life I accidentally licked my finger after it had come into contact with them, and the taste was extremely bitter. I think her lack of complaining was heroic. I can only imagine that she didn't want me to think I was causing her further discomfort by giving her meds.

Blind

"Diana is stronger physically and weaker mentally. I don't know what is happening in her brain, but I suspect the tumor is reaching the corpus callosum—the middle. In her delusional state, she talks about returning to work and taking a shower and having a beer and watching television. Even the watching television is getting to be impossible. I think she is going blind. Even with the shades up and the sun pouring in, she asks me to turn on the light. Much sadness there for me. Her hearing is sharp, but she can't interpret the sounds correctly." (From an e-mail message to my colleague Maureen McNulty, April 29, 1997)

As with other things, Diana never complained. She had a light touch, a gentle way of asking for things, and her saying, "Could you raise the shades?" when the shades were up and the room was filled with light, was so sad. Several days later, on May 3, I wrote in my journal: "We talk a little about her eyesight going. She is lucid. I stay with her a while longer, then go to bed so she'll sleep. I look over several times, and she is still awake—her eyes open and shut, open and shut. Then they are more shut than open. When I think she is asleep, I fall asleep."

Conversations about her failing eyesight were neither extensive nor emotional. So much else was going on with her recovery that losing her eyesight was less significant than the very real fact that she was alive. I did not know it at the time, but I think now that she was testing her eyesight that night by opening and shutting her eyes. It was typical of her not to discuss it. Or perhaps she might have thought I had already fallen asleep. I'll never know.

By the end of June, it was clear to me that she had lost her sight. I wrote to Maureen on June 28, 1997, "Diana is getting stronger, but [she is] still blind. We do physical therapy as much as we can, and she is sitting [up] for about 15 minutes a day. She gets discouraged about her sight and is worried about my going back to school in the fall. But overall life is good. Sleep is still a rare commodity." I want to emphasize that her discouragement was mild. I have no recollections of her ever fussing about it.

On July 2, 1997, I wrote in the meds log, "No sight—all gray." Two days later, on Marisa's birthday, I wrote to Maureen, "Yes, her ears are very sharp. She is sad about the loss of her sight. So am I, but I keep saying that if the eyes don't want to come along, it's their loss."

I took this rather tough approach to her blindness once it was definite that her sight would not I took this rather tough approach to her blindness once it was definite that her sight would not return. By the beginning of August, she was sitting in a wheel chair for one hour, and the excitement of her gaining strength and weight made her loss of eyesight almost insignificant. Again, what mattered most was that she was alive.

In November, Diana asked to visit an ophthalmologist to determine whether or not her eyesight might someday return. If not, she wanted to know what caused her blindness. We made an appointment with Dr. Egge on November 18, 1997. We arrived early and waited briefly in the car. It was a mild late autumn day. The air temperature was cool enough for us to wear jackets, but the sun felt warm on our face and hands.

Dr. Egge's waiting room was small, a tight fit for a wheel chair. We sat for ten minutes before rolling down the slim corridor to an examination room. We explained the reason for our visit before Dr. Egge examined her eyes. "The optic chiasma must have been burned by the radiation," he said as if he were reading a technical journal. I had thought for months that her blindness was reversible, but hearing Dr. Egge's pronouncement destroyed hope, and during this period, hope was the sunlight of our days.

He went on to explain that optic nerves run from the retina of each eye to the brain, and the ones closest to the nose cross over and travel to the opposite sides of the brain. The point where they cross is the optic chiasma (*chiasm* means *cross*) and all the optic nerves travel through this area.

When we returned home, we called Dr. Pierce, our radiation oncologist, and told her what Dr. Egge had said. Dr. Pierce confirmed the possibility that the radiation had hit the chiasma. Even though they had mapped the brain carefully, there was no way to avoid hitting at least some sensitive areas if they were to eradicate most of the tumor.

It would be presumptuous for me to describe what it is like to be blind. The closest I came to experiencing what Diana encountered occurred one day in the pool when she was working with Julie, our physical therapist. I closed my eyes for a moment. I, who have always had a strong sense of balance and a low center of gravity, felt as if I were in the ocean with strong waves buffeting me. I almost fell over. Diana, with her high center of gravity and with muscles weakened from eight months of lying in a bed, must have found it very difficult to stand, walk, or even to maintain her balance.

On January 7, 1998, Melanie Hughes of the Virginia Department for the Visually Handicapped visited us at our request. To quote from their literature, "The mission of the department is to enable Virginians with visual disabilities to achieve their maximum level of independence and participation in society." Melanie brought a cane with her, but unfortunately, Diana was not strong enough to walk unassisted, nor steady enough to tap the cane in front of her as we had seen so many blind people do.

On a subsequent visit, Melanie brought a three-dimensional layout of our room that she had built of cardboard and Styrofoam. She placed it in Diana's lap and moved Diana's fingers through the layout indicating the windows, doors, and beds. Melanie then asked her, "Can you point to the door?"

Diana thought for a moment then pointed to the wall.

"No, that's the wall. The door is to your right."

She sat on the bed looking very much like a three-year old who is aware she doesn't know the right answer and is mildly embarrassed. My heart went out to her.

Diana had always been spatially challenged, and once she was blind, she had difficulty remembering the position of the doors, the windows, the buttons on the radio, and the keys on our lap top computer. She could, however, remember the position of the plates and cups on the table.

Melanie's last visit was January 22nd, because it was clear to me that Diana was not strong enough to benefit from her help.

Soon after she had become bedridden in February 1997, to entertain herself Diana watched two videos we had taped off the television. One was *An Evening with Harry Belafonte*. We had attended a concert of his in 1967, and he was by far her favorite singer. The other tape was *Riverdance*, with the electric dancing of Michael Flatley, Jean Butler, and the Riverdance Irish Dance Company. Diana loved things Irish, especially plaintive Celtic music. I think she liked watching these tapes repeatedly not only because she liked the music, but also because they did not require intense concentration—this at a time when stress sent her into seizure.

One evening in December 1997, we both watched *Breakfast At Tiffany's*, which was dubbed for the blind with descriptions of the action. Even though I could see, I found the dubbed sections helpful in understanding the movie. I don't know that Diana had a favorite movie, but I do know she enjoyed this evening enormously. Audry Hepburn's portrayal of Holly Golightly was very like Diana, although Diana's romanticism was shot through with sound realism. She also liked Hepburn's compassion for less fortunate people.

Diana and I had had numerous arguments over the years about going to the movies—I wanting to get out on a Friday or Saturday evening, and Diana wanting to be at home to relax. If she did go out with me, she sat in cold silence through the whole movie. This night, however, we sat on her hospital bed, our legs dangling off the side, with our backs supported by pillows and cushions. For much of the movie, I had my arm around her shoulder, and from time to time she would lean her head against mine, or rest it on my shoulder.

As Diana's eyesight weakened during the spring of 1977, we turned from video to audio, and borrowed a few audiotapes from the Visually Handicapped Library in Richmond, sending off our request through the mail. Most of the books that we listened to during the summer, fall, and winter of 1997, however, we borrowed from the Fauquier Public Library in town. Many of these books were long—20 tapes or more—and some took us a week to finish. Diana loved books about travel, and we listened to Isak Dinesen's enchanting and spellbinding *Out of Africa*. She loved books about Britain, so we listened to *84, Charing Cross Road*, which is about a 20-year love affair between Helen Hanff, a New York Jewish lady, and Frank Doel, a proper English bookseller. And she loved Cynthia Helms's *Ambassador's Wife*, her account of being the official hostess in Teheran and an astute observer of Iranian culture, history, religion, and economics.

Diana listened to Noemi Emery's very long but engrossing *Washington: A Life*, a biography that included stories of his surveying parts of Fauquier County where we live. She loved current histories such as Robert MacNeil's *The Right Place at the Right Time*, including MacNeil's chance encounter with Lee

Harvey Oswald in Texas. She liked some of the 20th century classics, such as Steinbeck's *Cannery Row*. And she loved the mysteries of Patricia Cornwall that followed the adventures of Dr. Kay Scarpetta, Richmond chief medical examiner.

As I mentioned earlier, Diana loved our 1995 visit to Italy. Before going, she had taken private lessons to learn Italian. In March of 1998, blind and bedridden, Diana listened to Italian lesson tapes, pronouncing the words carefully and with great pleasure. One of the Sundays that month when Marisa visited, Diana asked her to put on the tapes. Marisa, of course, joined in and pronounced the words. Diana must have caught Marisa in a mispronunciation because she said, "I think you need to go to the doctor to have your ears checked." This was classic Diana.

Throughout her blindness, I was amazed that Diana did not complain more. I, and others, attributed her acceptance to her high threshold for pain and her life-long habit of not visiting her discomfort on others. I have no doubt that this is true. As I was writing this chapter, however, John mentioned Anton's Syndrome, which, in technical terms, is a failure of the brain to acknowledge blindness due to lesions in the occipital lobe. In other words, the tumor might have destroyed cells (much as mold damages bread) in the back part of her brain, thus preventing her from knowing that she was going blind.

For whatever reason, Diana accepted her blindness with grace and dignity.

A Day in the Life Of

The Room

When Diana left the hospital in February 1997, we had to decide which room in our house to place her in when she came home. We needed a quiet room away from the main traffic of the house and close to a bathroom. Some suggested turning the dining room into a bedroom—it would be close to kitchen and guests could readily visit her. Some suggested the den with a half-bath next to it and was across the hall from the kitchen. In the end, we chose the front north bedroom, upstairs and beside the front bathroom.

This was Marisa's room that I renovated in 1994 while listening to the 50-year anniversary programs of D-Day. The room measures 15 feet by 15 feet, and has an 8-foot ceiling. I had painted it a light green, a soothing color, with off-white trim.

Both doors in this room are wide enough to accommodate a wheel chair. The first door of the room comes in off the hallway, and the second door opens to the front bathroom. The front window looks out on to the street where we could see the Oldaker's house, and I was very grateful they kept it so beautiful because I rested my eyes by starring at it. The side window looked out onto Sarah Matson's white clapboard house. Sarah had died from cancer a year earlier.

The green room, as I now call it, was wonderful. It was large enough to hold a small group of people, large enough to move around in, and large enough to contain two single beds, a wing chair, a slant-top desk, a vanity, a mantle, a wardrobe, and an area rug. The large radiator beneath the front window kept it warm in winter, and the six-foot windows let in ample air in the summer. In early February, Diana slept in one of the single beds and I in the other. After several weeks, we replaced her bed with a hospital bed.

For Christmas, 1996, I gave Diana three photos I had taken in Europe and hung them in the green room when she returned from the hospital: a photo of the Ponte Vecchio in Florence; a photo of Diana in Florence which showed her smiling and happy, her hair swirled by the wind; and a photo of an antique doll in a store window in Strasbourg. A fourth picture, an oil painting done by John, hung on the wall beside my bed. And an old picture of St. Cecilia in an antique gray frame hung over the mantle.

I kept the room as beautiful as I could—for my own well-being as well as for Diana's. And we received many compliments on the room from guests. In a small way, it showed Diana that we cared about her.

A Representative Day

No two days during Diana's last year and a half were alike. She was recovering, she was declining; she was stronger, she was weaker; her medications were working, her medications were off. We ate breakfast every day, but some days I fed her, some days she fed herself, some days she ate a lot, some days she ate little; some days we chatted away, some days we listened to the radio—they were all different.

Because no two days were the same, we were never bored. The challenges, as great as they were, were always manageable on some level. We had something to look forward to each day—people visiting, going to the hospital for physical therapy when she was recovering, dinner, reading mail, making phone calls to the kids. We also had many memories to talk about.

Mostly, we had the present. When you think you're going to die, the present becomes very precious. We lived our days with as much attention as we had strength for. In fact, it was the attention we gave to our moments together that made life special—even when some of the things we were doing were heartbreaking.

From early February 1997, Diana was bedridden, and from then on she had only enough strength to get up in a wheel chair or for a brief walk to the bathroom. So the representative day I am creating comes from this, the last year of her life. In broad strokes, the following daily schedule is typical during the long period she was recovering, May 1997 to February 1998.

Typical Daily Schedule

6:00 A.M.	morning meds
8:00 A.M.	breakfast and washing up
10:00-11:45 A.M.	sponge bath and change clothes
12:00 P.M.	lunch and afternoon meds
1:00-3:00 P.M.	physical therapy three days a week, and on other days, reading mail, making phone calls to work and friends, listening to the radio or books on tape, and receiving guests on weekends and some week days
3:00–6:00 P.M.	exercises if no physical therapy
6:00 P.M.	dinner
8:00 P.M.	receiving guests, making phone calls to children, relatives, and friends
10:00 P.M.	evening meds, prayers, reading aloud from books, listening to the radio, or talking
11:00 P.M.	sleep

This schedule is much more orderly than it was in reality. For instance, sometimes she would stay awake for two or three days in a row. Other times, she might sleep for much of the day, and that meant we had to turn her at least every two hours to prevent bedsores. Regardless of whether it was a good day for her or bad, all days were very busy.

Don's Work

If there were a better job for me during this year and a half of taking care of Diana, I don't know what it would be. At the time, I was teaching writing at George Mason University and directing the Northern Virginia Writing Project, so typically I taught two days a week, prepared classes two days a week, and administered the project and did committee work the fifth day and for much of each weekend. When Diana got sick, my department chairs, Barbara Melosh and Rosemary Jann, excused me from all but necessary committee work. With the Internet hookup I had at home, I was able to keep in touch with the university and respond to memos and project business from home.

My administrative position directing the Northern Virginia Writing Project could have been a full-time job in itself rather than the equivalent of teaching one course. During the year and a half I took care of Diana, I had a reduced administrative load because my co-directors, Bernie Glaze and Bob Ingalls, along with my administrative assistants Karen Hickman and Mark Farrington, took on some, and at times, many of my duties.

Before Diana became ill, I was working a 70-hour week. After, I dropped it to 35 hours a week during semesters and 10 hours a week during the summer. The best part of my job has always been the flexibility of hours. During semesters, I was on campus about 16-25 hours a week, and was able to work the other 45 at home. In addition, I love teaching; working with students in the classroom and reading their writings during the night has always been refreshing for me.

After Diana became ill, I dropped my research and writing to a minimum. In fact, I was unable to revise one article slated for publication because I didn't have the time. Not many jobs allow you to postpone a portion of your work for a year and a half, so I will always be grateful for this job and the people who helped me out while Diana was sick.

Before I began the fall 1997 semester, Diana had become accustomed to my being home and was nervous about my being away. We had grown very close over the summer when she launched her recovery, and we both felt uneasy about being apart. We knew that if anything happened to me, the kids would take care of her, along with anyone we hired to help. I knew that placing her in a nursing home, regardless of the quality of the home, would be like placing her in the hospital. I would do anything to keep her at home.

Reading Aloud To Diana

There is something magical about a loved one reading aloud to you. Each morning, I scanned the *Washington Post*, and each week I looked through our two local papers for articles that might interest Diana. I skipped national and regional news because we caught that on the radio. But I did select more obscure topics, such as those dealing with technology and telecommunications, science and chemistry (her major in college), and, of course, medicine—especially articles on cancer. I stayed away from depressing and violent articles because of her low tolerance for stress.

The reading aloud she loved best, however, was reading from books, especially a book Brendan gave us Monty Robert's *The Man Who Listens to Horses*. She asked me to read each day, and I tried to fit it in, even if it were late at night. Sometimes, she fell asleep while I read, so I'd stop and pick up at that spot the next day. Sometimes, she added stories of her own, or I would ask her a question she could answer from her own life. For instance, after reading about Monty being beaten by his father, I asked her if her father had ever hit her brothers. These questions led to wonderful discussions.

Even though I am an English professor, I never considered myself a dramatic reader. I did improve, however, after months of daily reading—and Diana complimented me on it. I learned to relax my eyes, to move them ahead of the words I was speaking, and to place an interpretation in my voice.

Listening to the Radio

Even though we had a small television in the room, the pace of the shows was too frantic for Diana, and a number of times it caused her to seize. After a while, I turned the television on only for special occasions such as the funeral of Princess Diana.

I don't know how we would have managed if it had not been for the radio. In the morning, I turned on National Public Radio, and it stayed on for much of the day except when Diana was talking on the phone or talking with people in the room.

As I mentioned elsewhere, Diana was very intelligent, and the radio allowed her to grow intellectually. Several times she would correct the radio as when one newscaster cited the wrong name for one of the wives of Henry VIII, and another time when someone misidentified the lead song from *South Pacific*.

The radio not only kept us in touch with the world, it gave us something new to talk about. It also allowed us to carry on the demanding business of eating, bathing, and exercising with flexibility of attention. It gave Diana information she could give to people—which she loved to do. And, because knowledge can be power, even though she was bedridden, she was able to engage in the conversations carried on by those who could walk, see, and get about.

The following is a list of the programs we listened to throughout the day and sometimes throughout the night.

Morning Edition 6:00–8:00 A.M.
   We listened to this morning news program for the extended coverage it gave to feature stories and human-interest pieces. In many ways, we became very well informed on current events.

Diane Rehm 10:00 a.m. to Noon

This was the centerpiece of our day because Diane Rehm had important topics, expert guests, and informed callers. We noticed that high-quality talk show hosts attract high-quality callers. Rehm's topics spilled over into our conversations and gave us plenty to talk about. At times, I would leave this show on while Mittie or other hospice volunteers visited because they enjoyed talking with Diana about it. At other times, we would turn it off if we had things to talk about ourselves.

Afternoon Talk Shows Noon to 3:00 p.m.

We especially liked Derek McGinty's 12:00-2:00 p.m. talk show and were sad when he left radio for television. Derek was bright and adroit at moving the conversations forward. He also had the courage to say things we were thinking. Ray Swares from 2:00–3:00 p.m. had some great discussions on education.

Bluegrass Country 3:00–6:00 p.m.

Diana liked blue grass. Country music was so sad we would cry, and classical too serious and depressing. Popular music was either too reminiscent or too exciting. Blue grass was detached and soothing, and it never upset her.

Marketplace 6:00 p.m.–6:30 p.m.

Business news was interesting for us, especially news of the health care profession and telecommunications.

All Things Considered 6:30 p.m.–8:00 p.m.

The evening news.

Rebroadcast of Select Daytime Talk Shows 8:00–10:00 p.m.

We especially enjoyed having the chance to listen to shows we missed or ones we wanted to hear again.

The World and Fresh Air 10:00 p.m. to Midnight

Terry Gross interviewed authors and people of interest—including a few people we knew. The Canadian perspective on the news was interesting and different.

Midnight-6:00 A.M.

Several of the news and talk shows during the night originated from the BBC, while others were rebroadcasts of American daytime shows. We enjoyed the British and European perspective on the news, so we tried listening to a short wave radio but found the times of the broadcasts rarely coincided with times when we could listen.

The weekend schedule from NPR was different from the weekday schedule. It included *Car Talk* on Saturday morning, and we laughed and laughed at some of the problems people had with their cars, spouses, friends, and mechanics. It was as close to laughter therapy as we came. Diana loved Fiona Ritchie's hauntingly beautiful Irish music on "*The Thistle and Shamrock*" on Sundays from 5–6:00 p.m. I found this music enormously sad and often wept while listening to it.

Only once did Diana ask us to turn off the radio because of the content when Diane Rehm had a show on dying. Diana found it too depressing. The only time I switched to another station or turned off the radio was when it played sad folk music.

Phone Calls

It took over a year for Diana to absorb the fact that she might not be well enough to return to work. She was a manager in the best sense of the term, caring about people as well as the work they did for the corporation. She urged them to pursue advanced degrees and to take on tasks that helped them grow professionally. I could tell from the things her co-workers said about her that she was exceptional. In addition to heart, she had vision, the ability to look beyond the immediate, and frequently talked about the need to work on the Y2K problem long before it became a national issue.

Soon after she became ill, I went with her to clear out her personal things from her office. They were surprisingly few photos, a hand-held calculator, small gifts people had given her. Her fifth-floor, corner office with windows on two sides was sparsely decorated. Several months later, her friend Sandy Bodek would bring us five boxes of her things from her office—mostly books, papers, a few office toys, and photos of our children. She was elegant even in her office.

Diana managed work from home for the first weeks of her illness, and loved calling up her voice mail. The content of those calls gradually shifted from business to personal. People at work, in particular Sandy Bodek, Bruce Frietas, Janet Vaughan, Peggy Timms, Sharon Rose, Dottie Rosenberry, and Dave Johnson, were wonderful in keeping her involved. When she was confused, I know she left messages that didn't always make sense. Sometimes, she caught her mistakes in time to apologize and correct them. Sometimes, she would listen to the same message for several days. Other times, she knew immediately that she had heard it before.

Dave Johnson, who replaced Diana although Diana did not learn of this until late in her illness, held several conference calls with her, each lasting over an hour with several people sitting in his office talking over the speaker phone. I listened in and took notes as best I could in case she wanted to refer to things later. Much of the conversation was technical. We were amazed at Diana's ability to remember details, to focus on the problems that had to be addressed, and the clarity of her mind. She did this without referring to notes or being prompted by me. And I believe her suggestions were valuable even though she had been away from work for a year.

It was very important to her that she remain involved. Even though she was a mother and wife, she also had a job, and it meant a great deal to her that she not lose it, that she not be cut out of the loop. The respect afforded to her by the people at Cable and Wireless was, in my estimation, extraordinary.

In addition to work-related calls, which we made mostly in the afternoon, Diana talked often to her relatives and friends. A few times they had problems that seemed worse than her own—for instance when she called her cousin Madeleine in Petersburg, Virginia, who was 95 years old, blind, and living alone. Another cousin, Virginia, was battling cancer as well, as was her cousin George. In these calls, she was very solicitous of them, spending much more time talking about their condition than her own.

And we talked to each of our three children every day.

The mechanics of her talking on the phone remained a challenge throughout her illness. At times, she was too weak to hold the phone, so I would hold it or cradle it on a pillow. Some receivers were too heavy so we bought a different phone, one with large numbers and a very light receiver. Unfortunately, her spatial intelligence was not strong enough for her to know where the numbers were, so after January 1997, she never dialed her own calls. We tried a speaker-phone, but only one person could speak at a time, and the delay involved between the time when one person stopped speaking and the other person began was disconcerting for smooth conversations. Our best system seemed to be Diana sitting up with her right arm supported by pillows, holding a light weight corded phone in her right hand, and my talking on a cordless phone so I could move about the room folding laundry, cleaning, etc. That way each of us heard the conversation clearly.

Because the cancer was directing her activities, and even at times her thoughts, Diana had little control over her life. Consequently, when she wanted to talk to people, I did my best to get in touch with them. Sometimes, we planned ahead and make lists of people she wanted to talk to, and at other times, we called people on the spur of the moment. Only a few times did I suggest that she call at another time.

Mail

Once, while visiting my aunt and uncle in Florida, my uncle stood up from the table and walked down the driveway to get the mail. "Let's go see who loves us," he said. Receiving cards and letters from people felt like love.

Mail for us came mid-afternoon, and I would read the cards and letters to Diana in our quiet time before dinner. Most days brought a card from someone, and if a lot of cards came one day, I saved a few to make sure she would have mail the next day. I did the same on Saturdays so that she would have something on Sundays. I'd say, "Oh, here's a card we didn't get to open yesterday."

Some cards were sentimental and flowery, while some were humorous. Some people wrote all over the card, squeezing in one last word. Others were merely signed, "Thinking of you." Some told Diana how special she was, others filled us in on recent events with children and pets. All were love.

Even though Diana was blind, I taped the cards to the wardrobe, and it looked like a bouquet of flowers. One card, with a picture of tulips, came from her colleagues at work and measured 28 square inches. Marisa taped it to the door leading to the front bathroom. Visitors would read the wardrobe, and Diana would hear the cards again. They were a constant reminder that people cared about us.

I kept all the cards—as mementos and for their return addresses. I regret that time allowed me to write back to only a few people, and these cards or letters I composed with input from Diana, at times jotting down her sentences verbatim.

Three colleagues of Diana's made a special effort to write. Janet Vaughn sent cards and long, typed letters. She wrote about work, people at work, her family, house, and neighborhood. Her letters were well written and often humorous. We re-read them many times, laughing each time. Peggy Timms sent at least a card a week with diagonal writing across every inch. She also wrote about family and sent photos. Through her cards, we watched the weekly drama of her children. And Maggie Lawver, who sent very warm, long, typed letters lost her husband during the year Diana was ill. Several months later, Diana, bedridden and blind, consoled Maggie for her loss. It was an exceptional call. When Maggie visited, Diana brightened up and smiled. As I have said elsewhere, we had never been ill, so being on the receiving end of such affection for the very first time was truly moving.

Cooking Meals

When Diana dropped to 80 pounds in March 1997, I knew I had to increase the fat in her diet. I also had to cook meals she would find irresistible. If she didn't like something, she never complained—she just didn't eat it.

My cooking history was spotty. Like some men, I made my mother's marinara sauce and boiled spaghetti until it was more or less done. My mother had been a mediocre cook at best, so my appreciation for good food was minimal. When I cooked for the family, I tended to follow my craving at the time rather than a recipe. I also followed a few erroneous principles that got me into trouble in the kitchen, one being that if a little is good, a lot is better. I once made roast chicken with Italian seasoning. I liked the taste of Italian seasoning, so I poured it on. The chicken turned green. Another mistake I made was thinking that if I cooked something for an hour at 250 degrees, it would take me only half an hour at 500 degrees. The chicken turned black.

In the years after our children went off to college, I cooked many of the week-night dinners, trying to recall my childhood favorites. I stayed away from the dishes Diana prepared well, but I rarely used a cookbook. At best, my food had a one-dimensional taste. For instance, when I made curried eggplant, I pretty much cooked everything all at once in a large skillet—onion, green pepper, carrots, eggplant, zucchini, canned tomatoes, and curry powder. I didn't understand how foods responded to quick heat, and I didn't understand how seasonings needed to be added at specific times—not just thrown in. As mediocre as these meals were, Diana praised my cooking and was grateful because her job and her commute were so demanding.

With this as my history as a cook, it was no wonder that people were concerned when Martha and Randy left at the end of April because I would be preparing all of Diana's meals.

The first thing I did was to remember what my colleague Bernie Glaze had said about good food that it starts with the best ingredients. When I shopped, I bought the freshest, most nutritious, and best-tasting food I could find. I shopped at our local gourmet grocery store, at a natural food store, and on Saturdays in the summer, at the farmers' market.

The second thing I did was to select the best cookbooks we had and add to them. We already had *Southern Living Cookbook*, Jane Brody's *Good Food Book*, Carol Field's *The Italian Baker*, and several of James McNair's cookbooks, especially one titled *Soups*. To these I added Barbara Tropp's *China Moon Cookbook*, and Patrick O'Connell's *The Inn at Little Washington Cookbook*. Marisa and Glen gave us Tom Lacalamita's *Ultimate Bread Machine Cookbook* along with a bread machine, and I began reading two food magazines—*Gourmet*, which John had given Diana as a subscription, and *Fine Cooking*. I then developed a month of menus, asking Diana for her favorite meals and organizing each of the four weeks around one or two meats so that leftovers from one meal became the mainstay of the next. I desperately needed this month of menus because I didn't have the time to make decisions each day about what we were going to eat. Menu planning and cooking also became a very enjoyable topic of conversation for us. I was surprised at how much Diana knew about cooking, and with her prodigious memory, I found her directions to be the same as those described in the cookbooks. After she lost her sight, meals became one of her few pleasures—and she would ask each morning what dinner would be. It was important to both of us that I knew.

Cooking got off to a rocky start. I burned three pots in the first month. I replaced them with a starter set of LeCreuset cookware, thinking iron was a little more forgiving. Some of the early meat meals were not delicious. I had been a vegetarian since 1978 and realized I could not cook meat and adjust the seasonings for Diana without tasting it, and I could not tell the effects of meat on mood, sleepiness, and nutrition without eating the same portions of meat that she did. So, I ate meat. I also had to learn to prepare meals quickly because cooking in the kitchen meant leaving Diana alone in the bedroom. Lunch was not a problem because I often had Carol, Mittie, a visitor, or someone from hospice to sit with her. Breakfast was not a problem because it took only about 15 minutes to prepare. Dinners, however, took an hour, and I cooked while someone was with her in the late afternoon, when she napped, or, as in most cases, I cooked as fast as I could as she listened to the radio. As it turned out, it was a good way to learn, and after a while, I managed to get everything ready quickly. I want to make it clear that what made it possible for me to become a successful cook for Diana was the appreciation I received from her and from visitors who ate with us. Diana showed her appreciation not only through words, but also by eating well and gaining back her full weight from 80 to 146 pounds in five months.

Eating Meals

From October 1996 to February 1997, Diana was able to feed herself. Then, for about six months, she was so weak that she had to be fed, and feeding Diana could take as long as two hours per meal or six hours a day.

    I cooked and prepared the meals in the kitchen, placed the dishes on a tray, carried them upstairs to the bedroom, and placed them on the bedside table. This was a wooden table on wheels made by Levenger that I rolled around to stand beside the bed or above it. I positioned it on Diana's right because I'm right-handed. It was difficult approaching her mouth from the other side of the bed when I held the spoon in my right hand because my hand was between the spoon and her face.

When feeding Diana, I used mostly spoons, but also forks, and, at times, I used my fingers if feeding her a sandwich. I used a 3 1/2 inch paring knife to cut the food into bite sizes. When Diana was particularly weak, I used the blender to soften the food—even the meat, adding broth or gravy to the blender. I never blended the whole meal together because all meals would then taste the same. She deserved separate tastes.

Diana was a slow eater even before she became ill. I would finish a meal, and she would be only half way through. When she was weak, she ate even more slowly, taking as long as five to ten minutes to eat a spoonful. I have to admit that at the end of dinner, after spending six hours during the day feeding her, I was tired. I had to learn to occupy my mind with conversation, listening to the radio, or talking to her even when she was unable to respond. I also had to stretch and do back bends.

She always noticed my attitude when feeding her. When I was tired or impatient, I would rush the pace of the feeding, and she would slow the pace of her chewing. When I was patient and loving, she would thank me. A few times, she would try to keep up with a faster pace and store unchewed food in her cheeks like a squirrel. I wouldn't find it until we brushed teeth afterward.

We used covered plastic mugs and flexible plastic straws for liquids, and alternated the food and liquids throughout the meal.

Because it took her so long to chew, I sometimes forgot what I had last given her. So I arranged the food on the plate in a circle. For instance, I would feed her chicken, then mashed potatoes, then carrots, and move in a circle from one to the other. If she were eating particularly slowly, I used a different spoon or fork for each item and placed it facing up or facing down to keep track. This may sound bizarre until you have spent six hours a day feeding someone, and then it makes sense. If it looked like it was going to be difficult for Diana to eat, I would eat something while preparing the meal so that I wouldn't be distracted by hunger or by feeding myself while trying to feed her. When guests visited, I would ask them to feed her so that I would get a chance to sit in the wing chair, feed myself, and relax.

About half way through the meal I would ask, "What would you like more of?" and she would give me priorities, such as: "More meat, a little more potatoes, and no more carrots." If possible, I fed her meds at the end of the meal so that she already would have something in her stomach.

During the late summer, fall, and early winter, Diana was completely blind but strong enough to sit up and feed herself. To sit up, I raised the head of the hospital bed as far as it would go, and Julie, our physical therapist, taught her to turn to her left and push up with her right hand and slide her legs and feet off the bed. Her left side was always the weaker because of the tumor being on the right side of the brain. In the beginning, she needed help, but after a while, she was able to sit up mostly on her own. It was a wonderful move and gave her a sense of independence. Once she was up, I placed two large cushions behind her, plus any pillows she might need to give her support. I covered her with whatever sheets and blankets she needed to stay warm, then slid the foot of the bedside table behind her feet so that it was in front of her.

On the right side of the table, I placed two plastic mugs with covers—one holding juice or water, the other coffee. In the middle of the table, I placed the bowls with the entree in them and a spoon beside them. I moved her hands to the bowl and told her what was in each one. In the beginning, I placed her food on plates, and that made it difficult for her to scoop the food onto the spoon, so I bought bowls and pasta plates that had rims against which she could push the food.

I also bought several covered dishes to keep the food warm, and brought them up to the room on the tray. Because it took

Diana a long time to finish a meal, I placed small portions in her bowls and plates, then replenished them with warm food as she moved through the meal.

Sometimes, she would be strong enough to sit up, but not strong enough to feed herself. At such times, I would sit on the bed beside her and place both our dishes on the table and eat with her, feeding her at her pace. I often placed my left arm around her shoulders, and she would rest her head on me. These were sweet moments.

Bathing

A bath began in the bedroom. I would slide off her pajama bottoms as she stood and transferred from the bed to the wheelchair, and then I would wheel her into the front bathroom, directly in front of the tub. I then placed a large towel on the side of the tub, and lifted her feet to rest her ankles directly on the edge of the tub. As I slid the wheelchair forward, her long legs folded into the tub. I then climbed into the tub myself, placed my hands under her armpits, and on the count of three, she stood, pivoted, and sat down in the bath chair with her back to the spigot. Then I helped her out of her pajama top.

I turned on the water to get the right temperature, then with the hand-held shower nozzle, I sprayed water on her back. She checked the temperature, and I adjusted it. I then gave her a shampoo, massaging her scalp (she loved this part), followed with conditioner that I left on as I washed her back and bottom. Meanwhile, she washed her front and legs. I washed her feet and the backs of her legs, and checked to make sure she was clean all over. I then rinsed her hair and to keep her warm wrapped a towel around her head, another around her shoulders, and a third around her legs.

To get out of the tub, we reversed the procedure—pivoting and standing, then sitting on a towel in the wheel chair. Getting out was riskier because I had to make sure I positioned her feet close enough to the side of the tub so that her long legs would enable her to sit back far enough to land in the wheel chair. I also had to make sure the wheels were locked. I then climbed out of the tub and backed up the wheel chair so that her legs slid back over the towel. When they reached her ankles, I helped her lift over the right leg, and then lifted the weaker left leg myself.

I used an electric dryer to dry her hair, and she would remind me that it was too hot when I came too close to her scalp. I loved drying her hair, moving the brush through it. By December, her hair was thick and full, and almost all of it had grown back. To find the surgery scar, you had to search for it because it was not readily visible. These were relaxed moments for us—warm shower, steamy bathroom, rhythmic motion of the brush, and gentle talk.

As everyone who attended her knew, she had beautiful skin, an olive hue, which I thought came from the Spanish who shipwrecked with the Spanish Armada in 1588 and mingled with the fair-skinned Irish. She said, only once, that she thought her olive hue might come from an eastern European influence. I don't know, but it was beautiful.

After her hair was dry, I slid deodorant under her arms and moved her wheelchair up to the sink where she brushed her teeth, somewhat guessing where to spit. I also washed her face with Clinique and applied moisturizing lotion. It's amazing that with all her meds, her skin didn't dry out. Her dark hair made it unnecessary for her to use eyebrow pencil.

Laundry

We were very fortunate to have an extra-large-capacity washer and dryer in the kitchen, rather than the basement. It was easy to pop in a load of laundry while waiting for something to cook. On an average day I did three to four loads of wash. Laundry was like breathing—it was something I did all the time without thinking about it. During spare moments, I folded towels.

I collected laundry by placing a large, bath towel on the floor of the bathroom, then threw washcloths, pajamas, sheets, towels, and pillow cases on it. When it had grown to a mound, I gathered it up, and carried it downstairs in my arms.

Diana was incontinent for about half the year and wore disposable diapers. I was constantly washing the towels we placed beneath her, and when she wet the bed beyond the chucks and towels, I changed the sheets. When she was continent, I changed sheets every two or three days, and sometimes, every day if needed.

I used a liquid detergent, liquid fabric softener, and bleach regularly, especially if she had wet the towels. I got to know the softness and size of every towel, for each one had its own character. Some were large and absorbent, and these, I placed under the chucks. Some were soft, and these, I rolled up to cushion her head. Smaller towels, I rolled up to place under her neck or under her arm to keep her elbow from touching the bed or pillow. As I mentioned elsewhere, she had no bed sores and keeping bony parts, such as her elbows, off the bed prevented them.

I should probably mention that I once washed the wool blanket in water that was a little too warm. I then told Diana, "I'm making a baby blanket."

Getting Out of the House and Back

Most of our excursions out of the house were for physical therapy, either at the hospital, in which case Diana wore street clothes, or the pool to which she wore sweats over a bathing suit. The five times we went to parties, she wore her dresses or slacks and blouses. Wherever we went, however, the procedure for getting out and back was the same.

We began by getting dressed sitting on the bed. Getting out of her pajama top and into a bra and blouse was relatively easy. Getting into her bathing suit was a little more difficult because it involved standing. I would get her out of her pajama bottom with one stand, and slide up her bathing suit with a second stand.

Getting on her sweat pants involved a third stand, and this I combined with the pivot to the wheel chair. We saved putting on her shoes until after she had made it down the stairs because her shoes caught in the carpet.

Once dressed and in the wheel chair, I wheeled her out of the bedroom and down the hall to the top of the stairs. There, I stopped and came around to the front of the wheel chair where I helped her to feel the banister so that she would know where she was. I then placed my hands under her arms and helped her to stand.

This was somewhat tricky because the stairs were behind me, and if she were to fall forward, I had to make sure I could rest her on the floor before we both tumbled down the stairs. Once she was standing, I kicked the wheelchair away from her, moved around behind her, placed my leg against her bottom, and moved back as she slid down my leg to sit on the floor. Because she had a lifelong fear of falling, I had to make sure she knew she was not near the top of the stairs. I asked her to sit in that position until I took the wheelchair down the stairs. I folded the chair to roll it past her, then wheeled it down.

When I got back up the stairs, I lifted her under her arms and inched her forward. She was able to move her right leg out front, and I helped with the left.

We repeated this motion until her feet were on the second step and her bottom was on the top. In December, 1997, she was able to inch down the stairs on her bottom by herself; it took her about ten minutes to make it down the fourteen steps to the landing, and then an additional three to the first floor. She needed help making it across the landing, but then continued on her own until her feet were on the floor. From there, I again helped her to stand, pivot, and sit in the wheel chair. There I put on her shoes and laced them up before placing her feet on the wheel chair rests.

I then ran out to the car, unlocked it, started it, and switched on the heater. Back in the house, I helped her pull on her coat, then buckled her into the wheel chair.

I rolled her backwards out of the front door, locked it behind us, and then tilted the wheelchair back to descend the two porch steps to the front walk. Halfway up the walk, I turned her around, opened the gate, latched it open, and pulled her up the two steps to the street, and the one step down onto the pavement. Moving backward, I pulled her beside the car and locked the brakes on the wheelchair. I then unbuckled her belt, helped her to stand, pivot, and sit on the passenger seat.

I lifted her legs into the car, slid her around so she faced forward, and buckled her seat belt. I then closed the door, wheeled the chair around to the back of the car, removed the footrests, folded the chair, and slid it into the trunk.

Once in the car, I gave us each a breath mint. Diana asked for them shortly after we began getting out, so I kept one box in the car and one in my coat pocket. Perhaps her sense of smell had become stronger when she lost her sight, thus enabling her to smell things I could not. I'll never know. I gave myself a mint as a reward for not dropping her.

Getting from the car to the hospital or someone's home was the reverse procedure: wheel chair out of the trunk, getting out of the car, pivoting to the wheel chair, buckling up, and wheeling into the building.

Returning home, however, was different. The two steps from the street to the front walk were steep, so I built a ramp out of plywood, with edges on the side so the wheels would not slide off, and wood strips down the middle to give me traction. I actually had to push against the chair as we descended the ramp backward, to keep us from careening down and into the boxwood. A few times, we descended quicker and rougher than I liked, and from Diana's point of view, precariously because she was tilted back, riding backwards swiftly. If it went well, I'd say, "That wasn't so bad, was it?" And she would say, "No, that was OK."

Once inside the house, I had two choices. If she were strong enough to ascend the stairs, I would get her out of the chair and pivot her to sit on the first step. She then inched up the stairs as I lifted her under her arms, one step at a time. After each step, I leaned over her to help her lift her legs, again, one at a time. Once at the top, I cheered and helped her move back away from the stairs so that she would be at ease. I walked back down, wheeled up the chair, and positioned it well behind her. I then pulled her legs and feet as close to her as I could, stood behind her, bent down, and, on the count of three, lifted her from under her arms to a half-standing position. I placed my knee under her bottom, shifted my hands under her arms and straightened her to a full standing position. Then I moved beside her, and, with my left foot, slid the chair behind her, moved to the front, and helped her to sit. It took enormous strength, determination, and courage for Diana to ascend the stairs this way, and she never once complained.

If she were not strong enough to ascend the stairs sitting down, I called our neighbors from across the street, David and Kay Oldecker—and whoever was free came over and hoisted the bottom of the wheel chair as I lifted the top, and we wheeled her up. Because she weighed close to 150 pounds, we often found ourselves panting by the time we reached the top.

I wheeled her into the bedroom where I unbuckled her from the chair, helped her to stand, and then, after pivoting, helped her to sit in the bed.

Before leaving this section, I want to recount two experiences we had. One sunny day in December, I wheeled Diana from the side of the car to the curb and then backed the chair to the curb until I could open the gate and set the ramp. When I returned, I could see the sun shining on her face—and even though she didn't say anything, I could see she was enjoying it. It was so cute to see her tilting her face up ever so slightly to catch the sun. I stood behind her for several minutes; neither of us spoke. Then I leaned down and rubbed cheeks with her. It was delicious.

The other time was when Pat Gould from Hospice was leaving the same time I was taking Diana to physical therapy.

By this time, we had the well-practiced routine I describe above. When we reached the sidewalk, Pat was ahead of me opening the gate—but she couldn't find the strap attached to the mailbox post, which held the gate open. I became so caught up in showing Pat where the strap was and how it hooked into the gate, that I let go of the wheel chair. We both turned around to see that Diana had rolled into the boxwood.

We both laughed the laugh of those in church who know they shouldn't be laughing, but can't help themselves. There was something very funny about a blind person rolling off into the bushes in her wheel chair. As I write this, I have a sense of Diana looking down at me as if I have a perverted sense of humor. All I can do is smile.

Foot Massage

Diana was never one for massage—neither a receiver nor a giver. But she did come to enjoy foot massages, and she let hospice workers, family, and friends give them to her.

Before she became ill, Diana never once had a massage. She was very private about her body, dressing modestly. She would hug you as part of a salutation or valediction, but she was not a touchy-feely person.

She spent a lot of her last year bedridden. Her circulation was always good, as far as I could tell, but she still needed to be exercised to prevent stiffening, bedsores, and a break down of the body.

We gave her foot massages on a regular basis. We propped her feet up on one of the bulkier pillows, and wrangled off her socks—wool, to keep her feet warm, the largest size I could find, washed along with all the other was—therefore a little snug on her size 9 feet. If our hands were cold, we ran them under the hot water in the bathroom sink. Then we squeezed lavender lotion into our hands, rubbed them together to warm up the lotion, and rubbed it on and into her feet, her ankles, and sometimes her calves. She was never emotive in her appreciation, but she was grateful, and we considered her falling asleep during a foot massage a very high compliment.

Cleaning the Room

Diana was allergic to dust and mold, so every morning after breakfast, and occasionally at other times of the day as needed, I washed the floor with an old washcloth. Even with the air filter running 24 hours a day, the floor still accumulated a layer of dust. I loved this simple act.

One day, while I was on my hands and knees washing the floor under her hospital bed, Diana said, "Are you using the good wash cloths?"

"No, this is an old wash cloth."

"It's not the same one you use on my face?"

"No, it's an old one. I keep them separate."

I could tell from the silence that followed that she didn't know whether or not to believe me.

Once a week, I also ran a wet rag over the windowsills, mantel, and picture frames.

I kept a vacuum cleaner behind the door and vacuumed every two or three days with the power nozzle on the rug and with the brush on the floors. I used the upholstery attachment to vacuum the wing chair, and the little bush to clean the picture molding and ceiling fan.

In late spring of 1997, Diana had more trouble with her allergies than usual, and when John came home, he said I needed to wash the white, cotton curtains—which I did. Her allergies improved.

We ran an air filter and humidifier continuously. I kept the temperature around 70 and the humidity between 50 and 70. The humidifier was important because it kept her mucus membranes healthy, providing a first line of defense against germs. She never once got a cold.

Blankets, Sheets, and Pillows

Diana was most comfortable with the room temperature between 70 and 74 and the humidity between 50 and 70. On days when she was immobile, she needed blankets and heavy sheets. On days when she was active, she needed a light sheet.

We used a lightweight wool blanket—lightweight because anything heavy actually gave her sores on her toes. We also used two cotton throws knitted by Elizabeth McLinden, mother of Karen, my administrative assistant. We had two heavy sheets that were unusually warm, and two light weight sheets that were cool. We used a combination of all of these to keep Diana comfortable.

We had three kinds of standard-sized pillows:

- soft, feather pillows, which we placed under her head or under her left arm. Because these were the softest, we could use them in places where her body was tender.

- Medium firm pillows, which we folded in half and placed under her hip and shoulder blades when we turned her.

- Large, fully stuffed pillows which we placed under her thighs/knees and calves.

We tried to keep her heels off the bed to prevent bedsores. We also placed these larger pillows under her elbows when she sat up to give her stability, and to keep her from listing to the left or right. When she was weak in the left side and blind, she would lean to the left and had to be propped up. When she spoke on the phone, we placed pillows under her right arm.

We had about 12 pillows in the room at all times and regularly used six when turning her—one or two under her head, two under her back, and one or two under her legs. When she sat up, we used the two large cushions, plus as many pillows as necessary to make her comfortable. We had an additional small pillow for the wheel chair. I tried to color coordinate the pillow cases so that we could grab a specific pillow without having to test it for firmness.

Changing Sheets, Towels, and Pillow Cases

When Diana was in the hospital in January 1997, I learned how to change sheets with her still in bed.

First, I unhooked the fitted sheet from one side of the bed and rolled it tightly toward the center of the bed. When Diana was well enough to help, she would reach across the railing and pull herself on to one side. When she was unable to move, we simply tucked the sheets under her. If she seized with even the slightest movement, I tucked the sheets very carefully.

Then I placed the clean fitted sheet on the bed and rolled it toward the middle, behind the sheet to be removed. If Diana were up on one side, she then released her hold on the rail and rolled over the rolled sheets onto the clean sheets. I then went around to the other side of the bed and pulled the sheets across, discarding the old sheet and smoothing out the bed.

In addition to the sheets, I also changed the towels, one that was placed under the fitted sheet and one over the fitted sheet, to keep her dry when she wet the bed. These were rolled with the fitted sheet to make a small hill for her to roll over.

The sheets had to be pulled tight because when she was bedridden for months, any wrinkle in the sheets might cause a bedsore in her body. At times when the sheets were not pulled tight, I saw the imprint in her back.

One person can change sheets this way, but it is easier with two. When Diana easily seized, I had to make sure her head did not move quickly, so one person lifted it gently while the other slid the sheets underneath.

I had one set of gray flannel sheets, one set of burgundy cotton, and two sets of white cotton—all 100 percent cotton because they breathed. Constant washing made them soft. The sheets had different temperatures—some warmer than others, and I tried to place the cooler sheets on the bed when the weather was warm. I also coordinated the colors—not for Diana because she was blind, but for everyone else who saw her. Making her look beautiful was relatively easy because she was, but making the bed look beautiful let others know she was worth the added attention.

Baby Monitor

Someone needed to be in the room with Diana at all times because there was no way to predict when she might need help. Responding to her requests, spoken or unspoken, made her feel loved, and feeling loved is what we all need.

When Randy and Martha stayed with us during February, March, and April of 1997, they took much of the day shift, and I took the night so that someone was in the room 24 hours a day. When they returned to North Carolina, I needed a device to allow me to hear Diana when I had to be out of the room.

Tracy, our daughter-in-law, suggested a baby monitor. I bought two in order to have two speakers. I placed the white, plastic monitor on the flat edge at the head of the hospital bed, and it was so sensitive that it picked up Diana's voice, breathing, and movements. I placed one of the two speakers in the kitchen and the other in the downstairs hall so I could hear her anywhere in the house.

I became like a parent of a baby, hearing the monitor without listening. I could carry on a conversation in the kitchen with guests while she was asleep, and when she awoke, I would hear her breathing change and knew I had about five minutes before she needed me in the room.

Sometimes I would be in the kitchen while she was listening to the radio, and she would say, "Donald, did you hear that?" and I would yell back up the stairs, "I sure did."

I once tried using two monitors, one in the bedroom and one in the kitchen so that Diana could hear me without my having to shout, but they squealed from feedback. I asked several people if there were such a thing as a two-way monitor, but there wasn't. A two-way monitor is a walkie-talkie, and that requires both parties to be able to press a button to talk. Because Diana was not strong enough to hold a walkie-talkie, much less be able to press a button, we were left with the baby monitor. But it was great. I loved being in touch with her that way.

Serious Talk

When I was in the kitchen, I listened with half an ear to the conversations Diana had with guests—keeping track of the time to make sure she wasn't tiring or nearing a seizure. I turned off the speakers if I knew that our next conversations would be private, or if I heard them steering in that direction.

I also kept track of how often she talked about her condition, about dying, or about the future of the children. If four or five days passed without serious talk, I initiated it. I would start serious talk with questions such as, "You look like you've had a few rough days. Are you seeing the same thing? What are you thinking about lately?" I tried to be somewhat rested during these conversations because I had to have the strength to listen carefully and not bring my own issues to the discussion. Diana deserved to be listened to unconditionally. I used the active listening techniques we had learned years ago from *Parent Effectiveness Training*, such as repeating her answer to make sure I understood it, allowing for enough silence so that she didn't feel rushed, and using expressions such as "Uh ha," to let her know I was still listening. Without making it formulaic, I also tried to ask *what* questions first ("What are you thinking of asking Dr. Maybach when he comes tonight?"), *how* questions second ("How do you think he'll respond?"), and *why* questions last ("Why do you think he would say that?"). I think this sequence made it easier for her to talk.

In the last year of her life, we had talked about every important issue we could think of. Had she lived, I'm sure we would have found an endless number of other things to discuss, but we left nothing important unsaid.

Closeness

Diana and I slept in our queen-sized bed from the time she had surgery in October 1996 until she went into the hospital in late January 1997. From then on, she slept in a hospital bed in Marisa's room, and I slept in a single bed across from her. Several times she asked me to crawl into bed with her—not to make love for she was never strong enough, but to be close. Her hospital bed did not have enough room for the two of us to fit comfortably, but we managed. I laid on my side, and she, of course, laid on her back.

When she needed emotional closeness, I asked her questions and responded as warmly as I could.

Sleep

Throughout her life, Diana never napped. "I won't be able to sleep at night if I do," she once said. In the months before she became ill, she would fall asleep after dinner sitting on the sofa in the living room. After she became ill, she took naps.

Sleep for a healthy person is a sign of tiredness, a chance to rejuvenate. Sleep for a sick person can also be tiredness, but it can also be a sign of decline—even approaching death.

In the summer of 1997, Diana would stay awake for two or three days in a row. I don't know if this was prompted by the drugs, by her body healing, or by fear that she might die if she were to fall asleep. During such periods, she would spend the night listening to talk shows on the radio as they were repeated from the previous day, and she would talk, and talk, and talk. Diana had never been a chatterbox with me, and I found this change delightful. Periodically, I would be quiet and glance over to see if she were tired enough to fall asleep, only to find her eyes still open. While she was awake, she also needed changing, feeding, and turning—no matter what time of day or night. I had no trouble going for two days without sleep, but I became tired on the third, and hoped she would be tired enough herself to sleep. She never stayed awake for more than three days.

I have always found it easy to fall asleep whenever and wherever I needed to. This was a blessing for taking care of her—for whenever she slept and I needed to catch up, I laid down, relaxed my body, let go of approaching thoughts, and was asleep within minutes.

When she declined in February of 1998, she slept more and more.

Physical Therapy

In late November and early December 1996, Diana lost strength in her left arm and developed a sore muscle in her left shoulder. She had used a heating pad, which helped, but the pain woke her at night, and by morning she was stiff. When she had her appointment with Dr. Dennis on Friday, December 6, 1996, she told him about her sore shoulder. He felt the muscle and said, "What have you been doing to yourself?" It was a gentle comment, but it still had a tinge of annoyance.

I felt defensive and wanted to say, "She hasn't done anything!" At the time, we didn't know what caused it.

Dr. Dennis diagnosed it as bursitis, and prescribed ultrasound, massage, and physical therapy three times a week for three weeks. I pictured a machine that spun your arm around to loosen it up. It goes without saying that neither Diana nor I had never been to physical therapy.

Our first appointment was the following Tuesday, December 10, 1996. When we signed in, I noticed that our therapist was named Julie, but no last names were listed on the sign-in sheet. The receptionist asked us to fill out an information form with the usual questions about the patient's condition.

We were sitting in Booth 1 when Julie came in drying her hands on a towel. She was short by our standards, wore a red sweater, and carried her shoulders straight. Diana was sitting in a chair beside the table, and I stood behind her. Julie asked Diana to describe the problem she was having with her shoulder, then evaluated Diana's range of motion, strength, and areas of pain, jotting down numbers on a chart. After this, she massaged Diana's left shoulder and back.

While massaging Diana's shoulder, Julie said, "I believe you know my parents."

"Who are your parents?"

"Eric and Jo Maybach." I was embarrassed because even though I had seen her once before, I didn't recognize her. She was the daughter of our family doctor.

Before leaving, Julie gave us homework—exercises to strengthen Diana's left arm and shoulder muscles. We returned the next day and reported to Julie that Diana's shoulder felt a little better. Again, Julie massaged her shoulder and back, then used ultrasound. As I understand it, the sound waves emanating from this machine stimulate the circulation of blood in the muscles at a level that is difficult to reach with massage. Diana told Julie that when she came to the hospital, the cold weather made her dizzy and nauseous. In subsequent sessions, Julie placed a hot pack on the table so Diana could rest her face on it and keep warm. I believe it not only helped her to relax, it also warded off seizures. Apparently, the cold weather caused her muscles to contract and thereby placed an overload on her sympathetic nerve system.

Before we left, Julie gave us exercises to stretch the trapezius muscles and instructions to keep a pillow under Diana's left arm to increase blood flow to the supraspinatus muscle. She also introduced us to the empty can exercise where you hold out your arm as if you are holding a can, then turn the arm around as if you are emptying it, and finally move the arm up and down to exercise the shoulder and back muscles.

We canceled our physical therapy appointment on the 16th of December because Diana did not feel well. We returned on the 18th and a pattern set in where Julie would give her a massage, roll the ultrasound head across her muscles, then give us new exercises to do. Diana always pointed out to Julie that these sessions made her feel better. Two days before Christmas, Diana attended physical therapy, but felt tired and nauseous as a result of the radiation treatments she was receiving at Fairfax Hospital. Fortunately, thanks to the physical therapy sessions, the pain in her shoulder had decreased, and her range of motion had increased about five degrees.

The day after Christmas, however, the effects of the radiation returned, and Diana felt so nauseous she had to take the antinausea drug Compazine, along with Tylenol III (Tylenol with codeine) to reduce the pain in her head.

Diana received her last radiation treatment on January 2nd and her second chemotherapy treatment on January 8th. She became weaker as she moved through January, and the slash, burn, and poison treatments took their toll. In the second week of January, I noticed a connection between her letting her head fall to the right side as she sat in the living room, and increased tightness and pain in her left shoulder and back. The knot in her left shoulder that formed in December returned by January 9th, and I was convinced that it was caused by her falling asleep sitting up and letting her head fall to the right side. On January 10th, she told Julie that she was concerned with weakness on her left side, weakness that Dr. Binder also had noticed before her second chemo treatment.

January 16, 1997 was the last physical therapy treatment Diana had with Julie before becoming very ill. On January 17th, we went to Dr. Dennis's office only to find the receptionist had erroneously scheduled us while he was on vacation in Egypt. Because of this, we did not have his approval for continued physical therapy treatments. Also during this period, Diana became weaker and more nauseous due to the radiation and fluctuations in her Dilantin levels.

Home Health

After spending a week in the hospital at the end of January, Diana needed to continue with her physical therapy at home to keep her left arm from becoming stiff. She was too weak to go to the hospital, and because Julie was licensed by the hospital for hospital work only, we called Fauquier Home Health to do blood work and to help her with physical therapy.

The Fauquier Home Health physical therapist was Jori, a tall, Swedish-looking woman with blonde hair and a reassuring manner. Jori's first visit was on Wednesday, February 5, 1997, and in this and subsequent visits, Diana had small seizures when Jori worked with her. Diana was very weak at this time, and because she wanted so much to do well, she became anxious and that caused her to have seizures. John told us that seizures by themselves were not a problem, but that over time they would weaken her. After a few visits, we asked Jori to stay in the living room and give us instructions on what to do with Diana. We would then go upstairs, do the exercises, and report to Jori. When Diana became even weaker, we decreased the exercising and told Jori that Diana wasn't strong enough for physical therapy.

Julie Comes to the House

Diana regained some of her strength during the months of May, June, and July. In early August, Diana mentioned having an earache, so on August 6, 1997, Dr. Maybach visited to look at her ear. During his visit, we told him we were really impressed with Julie's manner of working with Diana, and asked him if it were possible for her to come to the house.

Julie visited for the first time the following Tuesday, on August 12, 1997, at 5:00 p.m. after a full day of work. Even though she informed her supervisor, Barbara Stark, she visited not as a professional, but as a friend to work with Diana. She came twice a week, usually on Tuesdays and Thursdays, visiting 22 times until

Diana was strong enough to go to the pool on October 31, 1997. It is hard to imagine Diana making the progress she did if Julie had not worked with her during this period.

Diana had been gaining strength in June and July, although she was still bedridden. She was blind by early July, and her muscles were very weak from over six months of limited use.

Julie brought exercise sheets with her, which described strengthening routines that Diana could perform while lying flat on her back in bed—exercises such as:

knee bends
pelvic tilts
thigh relaxers
head rocks
arm reaches
fist tightening
quad sets
ankle bends
arm and leg strengthening exercises

More importantly, Julie brought an unshakable attitude that it was possible for Diana to get up and walk again. Julie's voice was strong and clear, and her descriptions of the exercises were precise and detailed. Julie showed me how to stand behind Diana and use my knee to help her to stand. Julie considered such movements quite simple, but we could not have discovered them on our own. Diana exercised every day, never once complained, and, like a child, smiled the cutest self-congratulatory smile when she accomplished something. I found myself cheering her on and actually yelling with excitement. These were truly happy days because there was hope in the room.

Julie mentioned that she had seen patients make remarkable progress with aqua-therapy, and said she thought the pool would allow Diana a greater range of motion because her body would be buoyed-up by the water.

At one point, Diana asked Julie, "What would I have to do to go to the pool?"

Julie said, "Safe transfer to and from the wheel chair."

Diana first sat in the wheel chair on July 23rd when John and I lifted her from the bed to the chair. We were jubilant, and Diana cried when she got back in bed because it was so hard to do. Later, she said she had gotten her right and left legs confused and said that if she had remembered to push on her right leg, she would have been able to help more. It was so like Diana to want to do things well. On August 2nd, she sat in the wheel chair for one hour. On August 8th, we wheeled her down the stairs to sit on the porch for half an hour. So, by the time Julie began her visits on August 12th, Diana was eager to become more independent and self-sufficient.

One of the first things Julie taught us was how Diana could roll on to her left side and, once the head of the hospital bed was elevated, push off with her right hand and left arm to come to a sitting position. Prior to this, I had brought Diana to a sitting position by kneeling on the bed with my right knee and sliding my right arm over her left shoulder, around her neck and back, then pulling her up. At first, she was too weak to get up without help, but as she exercised, her strength returned, and she was able to sit up on her own.

Julie then brought us exercises aimed at helping Diana to stand and walk, exercises that were challenging but achievable:

shoulder shrugs
chin tucks
leg raises
side tilts
buttock squeezes
arm rolls
static strengthening for the arms
shoulder blade squeezes
knee raises

Before she became ill, Diana exercised along with a television exercise program called *Body Electric*. From this program, she knew movements that made the physical therapy exercises Julie introduced easier to learn. Over time, I learned the sequence of the exercises and would use the sheets only to refresh my memory. I called out the exercise, such as "leg raises," and then adjusted Diana's position only if she needed it. I also bought an inexpensive exercise bicycle consisting of two pedals on a stand, and Diana would pedal for five minutes at a time. Once, when she finished, I asked her where she had gone. She said, "Downtown."

The period from August, 1997 to January, 1998 was a period of firsts as she regained her ability to do things for herself. It seemed that we were reporting new accomplishments every day, and I know that at the end of many of these days, we went to bed tired and happy. The following are some of the more memorable moments I noted in the meds log:

> September 15, 1997 Sit on the bathroom commode.
> The bathroom commode was behind the door in the front bathroom, at the foot of the tub. To get to it, I wheeled Diana to the bathroom, closed the door, and then moved the wheel chair as close to the commode as possible. Then we executed a stand and pivot move that was tricky because there was almost no room for me to place my feet beside the commode. This meant that I could not negotiate a side-to-side movement and therefore had to get her into just the right position before she sat down. There were times when my aim was not perfect, and I had to shift her a little to the left or right. For anyone who has had to use diapers and a bedside commode, sitting on a real commode for the first time in eight-and-a-half months is a triumph.

> September 16, 1997 Stand with walker.
> To help her stand, I leaned over, placed my hands under her arm pits, and lifted her with both my arms and

legs until she pushed down through her legs and stood. Julie had brought a walker that Diana used on this day to stand by herself for the first time.

September 18, 1997 Transfer to the tub.

I had mapped out a strategy to get Diana from the wheel chair to the tub where she could sit on the shower bench. I checked it with Julie and Barbara, and on the 18th, we did a dry run (pun intended). The following day, Diana took her first bath since January. We were so excited, so happy. We called Julie to let her know, and she showed up a short while later with a bottle of champagne and a bottle of sparkling apple cider in case Diana could not drink alcohol. It was a wonderful day. From then on, Diana had a shower and shampoo every two to three days.

October 6, 1997 Scratches nose with left hand and stands by herself with walker.

Diana's left arm had been paralyzed during March, so her scratching her nose with her left hand in October was significant. She did it spontaneously—and when we realized what she had done, we were very excited.

October 7, 1997 Walks four steps (with the walker).

These first steps with the help of the walker were so hard. Diana said her legs felt as if they had lead weights on them. I thought her weakness was a consequence of the tumor. Julie thought her weakness was a result of being bedridden—in other words, the muscles had all but disappeared from lack of use. I came to agree with Julie the more Diana's strength increased. Throughout October, Diana worked very, very hard to increase the strength in her legs so that she could become eligible for physical therapy in the pool.

The Pool

Warrenton Overlook Health and Rehabilitation Aquatherapy Center is located adjacent to the Fauquier Hospital, on what is known locally as Hospital Hill. On Friday, October 31, 1997, we rode around to the back of the building where the entrance to the pool is located, got out of the car and into the wheel chair, then rode through the two sets of doors into the pool area. The temperature of the air was 83 degrees, so our glasses fogged up immediately. Diana insisted on wearing glasses, even though she was blind. We never discussed it, but I imagine she didn't want to be seen as someone who starred into space.

She was delighted to be going to the pool, but she was nervous about the water. Considering she was blind and had been unable to walk, this is understandable. In dressing for the pool, I had helped Diana into her black, one-piece swimsuit, with sweats and coat pulled on afterward. When we got to the pool, I unlaced her shoes, slipped them off, peeled off her socks, helped her out of her coat and sweat shirt, then wheeled her to the swim lift, an ingenious chair which gently lowers the patient into the pool. I helped her to stand, slid down her sweatpants before she pivoted and sat on the swim lift, then slipped them off once she was sitting. When she was in the chair, we buckled her into a blue waist float.

Julie wanted me to accompany Diana in the pool to give Diana physical and mental support, so, wearing a swimsuit and tee shirt, I walked down the stairs and helped Diana off the submerged lift. The water was a warm 91 degrees, but for Diana who was doing very little moving, the water felt chilly. As Julie described it, muscle contractions create heat. Once in the water, Julie positioned her in a green, square-shaped float that Diana could hold on to, along with a yellow, plastic, inflatable "banana" around her neck to make sure her face wouldn't go under. The second day of aqua-therapy, Diana felt as if her feet were slipping, so she wore pool sneakers and two-pound ankle weights.

Diana walked in the four-foot section of the pool, then pedaled for about five minutes, holding onto the green float. After ten minutes, she felt cold, so Julie led her back to the swim lift and hoisted her out of the pool.

Once out of the pool, I helped Diana to stand and pivot into the wheel chair. Jenny Willits, Julie's assistant, had placed one moist hot pack on the wheelchair seat and one against the back. This was crucial because the air felt like ice after coming out of the heated pool. I then rolled Diana into the bathroom/shower. I positioned the wheel chair next to the shower chair that was in front of the showerhead, locked the wheels, and helped her to lower her bathing suit to her waist. I then helped her to stand and tugged her wet bathing suit down to her knees. She pivoted, and I lowered her on to the shower chair. I used the hand held spray to give her a shampoo and shower, rinsed her hair and body, then dried her off before slipping on her underpants and sweatpants. When she stood, I dried her bottom and pulled up her pants before she pivoted to the wheel chair. There, I dried her hair with an electric dryer we had brought from home. Finally, I helped her into her bra and sweatshirt before wheeling her out to the pool area to put on her socks and shoes. All this took about 45 minutes.

Diana was able to increase her time in the pool from 10 minutes to almost an hour. Among the pool exercises she performed were the following:

biking
marching in place squats
push downs with barbells
step-ups onto a red plastic box
wall push ups
walking back and forth the pool in various depths of water
    using a blue, styrofoam float-board
side steps and hip abductions

Julie was right. Diana's progress was dramatic once she began aqua-therapy. After one month, she was walking 160 feet in the pool.

Here are some of my notes from the meds log of things Diana accomplished at home during this period:

> November 11, 1997 Goes down stairs on her bottom.
> Julie had taught us how to get to the top of the stairs and lower safely to sit on the floor, and this day, Diana went down the whole flight of sixteen steps sitting on her bottom.

> November 12, 1997 Walks to the bathroom
> Diana walked from the bed to the front bathroom, with my holding her by the left arm and guiding her. Even though she was always graceful, even in a fall, I had to be there in case she had a weak spell or tripped.

> November 20, 1997 Walks to and from bathroom and washes hands standing at the sink. Stands alone.
> This was somewhat tricky because she had to lean over the sink to wash her hands, a position which shifted her center of gravity. She had gained enough strength to stand by herself and hold her weigh—at this point about 145 pounds. This was a major accomplishment.

> November 21, 1997 Two walks to and from bathroom, a heavy workout in the pool, and then sleep at 5:00 p.m.
> Her strength was increasing by the day, and after the heavy workout in the pool, she was exhausted.

> November 26, 1997 Walks to shower. Three bathroom walks.
> Walking to the shower meant we didn't have to use the wheel chair to make the transfer to the shower chair.

November 27, 1997 Two steps down on stairs.

After descending the stairs sitting on her bottom, she asked if she could stand and walk down the last two steps. I helped her to a standing position on the landing where she inched herself forward until she could feel the step. She then faced the railing and lowered her left leg first, then her right, and repeated it until she was standing on the floor. It was a great day.

December 3, 1997 First day without the use of a bedside commode or bedpan.

This was the first time she was strong enough to walk to the bathroom each time she needed to use the commode. I kept the bedside commode in the room for a few days, then removed it to the master bedroom. Its absence from sight was a sign of progress. During this period, her workouts at the pool were rigorous, and she gained confidence in her ability to walk back and forth to the bathroom.

December 17, 1997 Walks up four stairs.

In the pool, Julie had been showing her how to step up onto the plastic box that lay on the bottom of the pool. Because she was buoyant in the pool, she could perform this exercise without having to hoist her whole weight. In her visits to the house, Julie had shown Diana how to do the same exercise on the steps just outside the bedroom. Two days earlier, Julie had shown her how to step up one step. It was a demanding exercise. On this day, Diana kept going and climbed four steps before inching back down.

December 28, 1997 Walks down stairs by herself.

All sixteen steps. This was cause for great celebration.

January 5, 1998 Walks up stairs after pool.

On this day, Diana had walked down the stairs to get to the pool, then, after a full workout at the pool, came home and walked up the stairs. She did not set out to walk up the stairs—just a few steps. Then as she climbed, it became obvious she had the strength to continue. She was smiling, and I was cheering. It was a great day. If I had to pick a day when her recovery was the strongest, it would be this day or around this time.

It is worth noting that one piece of equipment that we used at home to reduce the pain of Diana's sore muscles proved to be quite helpful. It is called a TENS machine, which stands for Transcutaneous Electrical Nerve Stimulator. It is similar to the more powerful machines used in the hospital and functions when you place the four adhesive electrodes around the sore muscle and allow a small amount of current (nine-volt battery) to pulse into the muscle. Because the muscle relaxes and no longer hurts, the patient can stretch and exercise it, and this assists in its healing. Julie brought this machine to the house on a 30-day trial basis, and afterward our insurance purchased it for continued use.

Julie Lists

In October, when Julie asked Diana what she wanted to accomplish, Diana said she wanted to be able to type, that is, to learn the keyboard so that even though she was blind, she could still do her work. Because work meant so much to her, in a healthy sense, she wanted to continue long after everyone else realized she would never return. She wanted to type so that she could write the documentation for billing programs they had developed at Cable and Wireless.

She also wanted to memorize the radio so that she could play it herself. We tried this several times. We placed it on the bed beside her and positioned her fingers on the buttons-the on/off button, the tape play button, the stop button, and the volume dial. Diana found it very difficult to remember the position of these buttons. Because she had very strong verbal intelligence, she had no trouble with her verbal memory, often correcting the announcers on the radio. She once corrected an announcer for mentioning the wrong king in renaissance England. She also corrected an announcer for citing a song as belonging to the wrong musical. But the knobs, buttons, and dials on the radio stumped her. She never did learn the radio.

Several months later, we did a second Julie List as we called it. This included the following:

1. walk up and down stairs
2. walk by myself safely
3. write (readable prose)
4. type up a project notebook for work
5. inventory the dolls

I added the last one because I wanted her to finish giving us information on the origins of the dolls in her antique doll collection. Before she died, John's friend Bryon had tagged 11 dolls, and in a notebook wrote a brief description of each doll with an explanation of how Diana had acquired it.

Her first priority, however, was to walk safely and by herself. Her second was to return to work. By the time she had dictated the second Julie List, she knew she was irreversibly blind—yet she still wanted to return to a mobile, productive existence.

Diana never talked about goals she might have for herself and never made lists for other people—what some called Honey Do Lists. She thought things through and then told you what she wanted done—often in a light, gentle manner tinged with a determination that let you know she was serious. She also let you know you could do it—although it might be a sizable stretch.

She worked very, very hard at learning to walk—and never showed discouragement. As with other things, you never got to see the scaffolding, the work behind the scenes, the turmoil or conflict within. If there were any, she kept it to herself.

Julie

To be complete, this section must contain a description of the exceptional person Julie was for us. From August 1997 until Diana's death, Julie directed Diana's recovery and brought with her, to our home and to the physical therapy sessions at the hospital, a conviction that Diana could walk again.

Julie visited our home over 22 times without compensation before Diana was strong enough to go to the hospital for aqua-therapy, and countless times after her decline. By any standard this is an enormous act of generosity. She also called us to check up on Diana's progress, answered our calls and questions, and loaned us equipment such as canes and walkers that made it possible for Diana to walk again.

When Julie first visited in August, she became aware that Diana was blind. To get a sense of what Diana might be feeling, Julie walked around her own house wearing a blindfold.

One cold, rainy day, as we were getting out of the car for aqua-therapy, Julie showed up the curb with an umbrella. This may sound like a small act of kindness, but when we were struggling with so much, it felt great.

When Julie worked with Diana in the pool, she anticipated Diana's pacing and ability and had the next exercise ready for Diana to move into. This made not only for a strong workout, but also gave us the message that this time was precious and not to be wasted.

At the end of November 1997, Julie's rotation at the pool ended, and our physical therapist became Jan Anderson. Jan, too, was a wonderful therapist, and Julie briefed her on our progress and kept in touch with Jan and us as we began a series of six visits to the physical therapy section of the hospital to supplement her aqua-therapy.

One day, I pulled a muscle in my back, helping Diana to stand. Julie noticed my stretching as she was talking to Diana and later arranged for me to receive several physical therapy treatments at the hospital. If Julie had not caught this problem early, it may have developed into an injury that would have prevented me from taking care of Diana. Julie, Jan Anderson, Jenny Willits, and Barbara Stark were responsible for my staying healthy during this period.

At one point, Diana said, "I wonder if the other Maybach children are like Julie or if they are mere mortals?"

Someone once said of Robert Kennedy that when he walked into a room, everyone appeared to be in shades of gray while Kennedy was in color. Julie has the same ability to light up a room.

We were incredibly fortunate to have her come into our lives.

Good Times and Getting Out

Diana was verbal; I'm visual and kinesthetic. When it comes to touch, I love it—and almost crave it. I communicate through my hands as much as through words. Diana communicated mostly through words.

We had many an argument over the years about back rubs. Whenever I asked for one, she would decline or give one with great reluctance. I don't recall her ever asking for a back rub herself. Early in our marriage, she would ask me to brush her hair, which was a reminder of the affection of her grandmother, and I enjoyed doing that for her. In fact, in the last months of her life, I found myself running my hand through her hair for twenty or thirty minutes at a time.

After many years of arguing about back rubs, I learned that some people are givers of back rubs, some are receivers, some are both, and some are neither. Diana neither liked giving nor receiving, and I liked both.

Diana's perversity played a role in the back rubs. She knew how much I craved them, and anything I really liked, she thwarted or pretended didn't exist. She would say, "I just don't like them, that's all." They weren't a big deal for her, but they were for me.

I think part of their importance came from my not being held as a child. I have no recollections at all of my mother ever holding me, and in the 1940's, men didn't typically show physical affection to their children. I believe the clinical name is touch deprivation. We actually met a couple who taught at Mason who had gone to a conference for touch-deprived people, and one of the exercises they were introduced to was to take care of the other person totally for 24 hours—which meant helping them to bathe and eliminate as well as eat and move. When I heard this, sometime in the late 1970's, I was amazed—even a little shocked. I couldn't imagine being so intimate with someone. But I was also drawn to it. Diana and I never attended a touch deprivation conference, but I thought of this often during her illness when I did take care of her totally.

The few times during our marriage when Diana consented to give me a back-rub, she moved her fingers as if she were touching raw eggs. I don't think she felt repulsed by touching my back, but I had reason to interpret her movements as if she were. She would rub more with the tips of her fingers than the palms of her hands, like a spider hopping across a warm stove.

You can imagine the surprise, then, when she offered me a back rub several times in her last year. She sat up in bed with her legs off the side, her back propped up with pillows resting against the rail. I sat next to her, and with her right hand, she rubbed my back. These back rubs were identical to all the others she had ever given to me, but they felt great.

I doubt that Diana enjoyed the physical sensations of giving me back rubs during this last year, but I do know she had a sense of peace about her over the issue. She volunteered back rubs, and this in itself was a resolution. I should also mention that there were times when she was unable to sit up, and she would still offer a back rub. In addition, she could tell if I were tired by the sounds of my feet on the floor—and she would say, "Would you like a foot rub?" I would slide the chair beside the bed and rested my foot beside her hand. I would then drip lotion on my instep, and she would rub it in. She usually had enough strength for about five minutes although never admitted she was too tired to continue.

I often say of her last year, "She gave when she had nothing to give." These foot rubs are one of the things I think of.

The Baby Showers

Marisa and Glen called us Monday morning, November 24, 1997, at 6:30 a.m. to tell us they were headed into Sibley Hospital in Washington, D.C. Marisa herself was born in Washington, and we noted that our second grandchild would be born in the nation's capital. As soon as we hung up the phone, there was no question that Diana was determined to go into the city to see the baby.

The day was sunny, cold, and windy. It took us about an hour, and we arrived at Sibley late that morning. Marisa was having back labor because the baby was facing her back when she needed to be facing her front. Because of the pain, she requested an epidural, even though she and Glen had gone to a series of Lamaze natural birth classes.

Glen's parents, Jo and Bill Faunce, were also there, so we went to the cafeteria for lunch. When we returned, we were allowed in to see Marisa.

"You lied about there being no pain," Marisa said to Diana. "You said it didn't hurt."

I had been present when Marisa was born with natural childbirth and I knew that Diana was not experiencing pain. I felt defensive about Marisa's comments, and told her she just needed to breathe. I don't think I appreciated the amount of pain that back labor could produce. In retrospect, I think Diana had a very high threshold for pain.

By early afternoon, Marisa was dilated only about three centimeters, and the nurses were predicting she would deliver around six or seven that evening. We knew Diana didn't have the strength to stay up that long with no assurance that the baby would be born even then. So, we came home, and went to physical therapy in the pool where Diana received a very good evaluation.

Glen called us after we got home to say Madeleine Diana Faunce had arrived. We were warmed that Marisa and Glen had decided to give Diana's name to Madeleine as her middle name.

Diana saw Madeleine for the first time three days later when we went to Marisa's for Thanksgiving. Marisa placed a large black and white pillow on Diana and placed Madeleine on it, and just as Diana had done when she first held Nicholas, she became quiet, moving her long fingers over the baby.

When we ate dinner, Diana said grace and talked about how grateful she was to be able to hold Madeleine.

In the following months, Madeleine and our first grandson, Nicholas, visited often and lovingly. One time Marisa placed Madeleine on Diana's bed, and Diana sang, "Hush, little baby, don't you cry…" in her plaintive yet strong voice. A while later, Madeleine, Diana, and the cat took a nap together on the same bed.

During this period, many people told me that they thought Diana was fighting to stay alive to see her grandchildren. I think she would have fought to stay alive to be with her own children even if Marisa and Tracy had not been pregnant. But they were, and the joy and sense of closure Nicholas and Madeleine brought her were beyond measure.

A Trip to the Dentist

Diana had been concerned about her teeth throughout her life and took excellent care of them, using both water-pick and floss. She kept her water-pick on the counter beside the kitchen sink because the shelf above the sink in her bathroom was not sturdy enough to hold it. She used the water-pick at least once a day—usually at night before going to bed.

On December 16, 1997, Diana, Carol, and I drove to Fairfax to our dentist, Dr. Ha. Dr. Ha's office was on the second floor of a strip mall without a handicap entrance or elevator. Carol and I lugged Diana's 144 pounds in her wheel chair up the 24 stairs, my pulling and Carol pushing from beneath. I was so afraid of not being able to get to the top that I pulled her up as quickly as I could. When we got to the top, my heart pounded in my chest. Because Diana was blind, I don't think she thought about what would have happened if we had lost control of the chair.

After a momentary wait in the reception area, we wheeled Diana back, and I helped her to transfer to the dentist's chair. Dr. Ha is a diminutive Korean woman with a sparkling wit. From the reception area, Carol and I could hear Dr. Ha and Diana laughing. Diana spent two hours in the dentist's chair and survived without a seizure.

Before we left, Dr. Ha recommended an electric toothbrush that I bought a few days later, and it was wonderful. The spinning brush allowed me to clean areas I was not able to reach with a regular toothbrush, and I'm sure her mouth and teeth felt much cleaner. In addition to the medications, Diana was drinking a variety of fruit juices that left a sticky film in her mouth. The electric toothbrush took care of that.

Diana was pleased to be out that day, and came back in good spirits.

Sharon Rose Party December 20, 1997

Sharon sent a dozen of some of the most beautiful white roses to Diana when she was awaiting surgery. Throughout the year, she visited several times, and then invited us to a party along with Sandy and Bruce, Dottie and her husband Rob, and Bob Roger and his wife Michelle.

The party was scheduled to begin at 5:00 p.m. in Sterling, about an hour's ride from Warrenton. That meant getting into the car by 4:00 p.m., which meant getting into the wheelchair by 3:30 p.m., which meant getting dressed around 3:00 p.m., which meant a shower around 2:00 p.m. In December, she was getting stronger because she was working harder and harder each time she went to physical therapy in the pool. It was a good time despite her blindness and occasional seizures.

We followed the usual routine for getting out, and after her bath and shampoo, I washed her face with Clinique and applied moisturizing lotion. I thought it was amazing that with all her meds, her skin was not dry. Her dark hair made it unnecessary for her to use eyebrow pencil, although she did when she was well. I also helped her to apply lipstick, light enough that it would not come off on my clothes when I transferred her in and out of the wheel chair.

She donned a new bra that I had bought in the local department store because she had gained enough weight to outgrow her old ones. She slid on a white blouse, underpants and slacks, then socks. We saved slipping her shoes on her feet until after she had made it down the stairs.

On the way to Sterling, we talked about the people she had worked with, especially the ones we would see at the party—a light chatter—and the one hour ride passed quickly. When we arrived at Sharon's, Bruce and Sandy were also pulling up, and Bruce helped me carry Diana in the wheelchair up the front steps and into the house. After I helped her out of her coat, and after we said hello to everyone, I wheeled her around the first floor, describing the rooms as we went. This describing had become a habit by now—I felt as if I had become her eyes. Sharon's house was stunning. The Christmas tree shimmered with tinsel and lights, candles dotted the furniture and mantel, and the vaulted ceiling gave it a sense of graciousness. We wheeled into the den and out onto the porch where it was cold. When we returned to the large kitchen, we talked to people as Sharon finished preparing the chicken cordon blue.

The conversation and light banter during dinner were the most warm hearted I experienced in the year-and-a-half of her illness. Diana was incredibly witty that night as she paused before delivering one-liners with perfect timing. I know now that as she paused, she moved past the stereotypical thinking to make original statements.

We left at 10:00 p.m. Bruce again helped us down the stairs, and I helped Diana stand and pivot into the car. We were both very happy during the ride home. We talked about the party, then fell silent. After a few moments, Diana said, "I was really funny tonight, wasn't I?" Her voice was proud and humble, pleased with herself, but not bragging. She was also surprised, and there was a wonderful sweetness in her.

I replied, "Yes, you were very funny tonight." We rode much of the rest of the way in silence, very, very content.

When we arrived home, it was after 11:00 p.m., and I could see a light in the Oldacker house across the street. David and Kay had helped us up the stairs innumerable times after our trips to the hospital, sometimes coming out when they saw the car drive up. Diana wanted me to call them to help us into the house. I told her we could make it into the house by ourselves, and I would call them when we got in. Once we were in the house, I called David. This was the first and only time he wasn't able to help us because Kay was babysitting and David didn't feel comfortable leaving Harrison alone at night. I told him not to worry, that we were able to make it up the stairs by ourselves.

Diana didn't have the strength to walk up the stairs, so she sat down and inched up backwards. Once up, I wheeled her into the bathroom in front of the sink where she brushed her teeth and washed her face. The evening had left us tired but happy. As I watched her wash her face, I was aware that there was no obstruction to my vision. I could see Diana for who she was, and my gaze on her was relaxed and gentle. The love her friends gave to her and the laughter of the party had shaken any selfishness out of me. I looked at her with love, and she felt it. "You're taking good care of me tonight," she said.

I wheeled her to the bed, helped her out of her clothes and into her pajamas, gave her her evening meds, and lowered the head of the bed. I kissed her goodnight and climbed into my own bed. We talked briefly before I turned out the light. I believe it was the happiest she had been in over a year.

Things Spiritual

Lovingkindness

The year before Diana became ill, she would eat breakfast sitting on the swing on the back porch, looking out over our deep green yard, the fields, and the rolling hills beyond. When she finished breakfast, she would read a book a friend had given me by Sharon Salzberg, *Lovingkindness: The Revolutionary Art of Happiness*. Sharon is co-founder and senior instructor of the Insight Meditation Society in Barre, Massachusetts, and a practicing Buddhist meditator for over twenty-five years.

Lovingkindness is a wonderful book about opening your heart, facing the fear of intimacy, and cultivating love, compassion, joy, and equanimity. Sharon sprinkles the book with stories from her own life and from many cultures in a gentle, entertaining way. Here is one story pertinent to Diana's situation:

> "I was in a bad car accident in the late seventies. I arrived at Insight Meditation Society on crutches to teach a long retreat and I was having difficulty getting around. That was the year His Holiness the Dalai Lama came to visit. The preparations for his visit were intensive, because

we had to arrange a great deal of security for this man who is considered a head of state. Our peaceful, rural retreat center became a stronghold. Pleasant Street was barricaded off, and state policemen patrolled the roof with guns. There were video cameras and a lot of excited activity. I was feeling dismal on crutches, especially when I ended up in the back of a huge crowd waiting to greet the Dalai Lama when he arrived. The car with His Holiness in it pulled up at last and was greeted by the cameras, the people, and the armed policemen. The Dalai Lama got out, looked around, and saw me standing way in the back of the throng, leaning on crutches. He cut straight through the crowd and came up to me, as though he were homing in on the deepest suffering in the situation. He took my hand, looked me in the eye, and asked, "What happened?"

It was a beautiful moment. I had been feeling so left out. Now I suddenly felt so cared for. The Dalai Lama did not have to make the pain go away; in fact, he could not. But his simple acknowledgment, his openness, helped me feel included. Every act can be expressive of our deepest values." (Lovingkindness, Salzberg 2002, pp. 112–113)

A number of visitors felt shy about Diana's illness and didn't know how to approach her. Diana would reach out her hand to greet them and carried on conversations that focused not on herself, but on other people. When she was unable to greet them, I tried to make them feel comfortable, giving them something to do or including Diana in as much of the conversation as possible. I tried not to talk about her as if she were not there just because she was blind and bedridden.

Lovingkindness also includes twenty-three exercises aimed at teaching us how to develop universal love not only for people we love, such as benefactors and friends, but also for people we consider neutral or difficult. Instead of thinking of people through old thoughts and animosities, Sharon has the reader direct "lovingkindness" phrases toward them, phrases such as:

"May you be free from danger."
"May you have mental happiness."
"May you have physical happiness."
"May you have ease of wellbeing."

The result of reiterating these phrases is that we change the way we think about the other person—and we open our hearts to them. It is a healing of our emotional lives that diminishes our feelings of isolation, awakens compassion for other people-even those who have hurt us—frees us from self-created suffering, and teaches us to trust our instincts.

Before Diana's illness, when she was reading Sharon's book on the back porch, I would come outside to sit with her, and she seemed peaceful. She did not tell me what she was thinking, and we never discussed the book, but I think she read most, if not all of it, and I think she was practicing the exercises. She probably designated me as one of the "difficult" people.

During the summer of 1997, I ordered *Lovingkindness: Meditation*, two tapes that were based on the book and included meditation exercises involving lovingkindness. The tapes were read by Sharon, and her calm yet expressive voice was very soothing. Diana asked me to play these tapes in the late afternoon or later at night, and sometimes we fall asleep to them, and the tapes would run until morning. When Sharon's second book, *A Heart as Wide as the World*, came out in 1997, I bought it and read it aloud to Diana, making it to page 47 before she died.

We did not discuss the books or tapes much—I think we were lost in our own thoughts most of the time. Right now, I wish we had because I don't know what Diana thought about them or how much they influenced her extraordinary love for people in the last year of her life. I think her heart opened in January 1997, and her generosity was evident long before she listened to the tapes.

What I remember from these books and tapes is that lovingkindness is genuine love, without the extra baggage that so often accompanies love. In many ways, this is a tough practice because it does not allow for sloppy thinking or actions. At one point, Sharon writes:

> "In order to live with integrity, we must stop fragmenting and compartmentalizing our lives. Telling lies at work and then expecting great truths in meditation is nonsensical. Using our sexual energy in a way that harms ourselves or others, and then expecting to know transcendent love in another arena, is mindless. Every aspect of our lives is connected to every other aspect of our lives. This truth is the basis for an awakened life." (*Lovingkindness*, Salzberg 2002, p. 34)

I also remember that Sharon advocates a return of love for hate—that hating someone back for hating you doesn't work. The only way to break the cycle of hate is to love. "Return love for hate," is how I phrase it in my mind, and it works for me.

Diana was never interested in Buddhism or my practice of meditation. She did like the lovingkindness practice described by Sharon Salzberg, and my guess is that it strengthened her own natural inclination to love people. When she learned that Mittie had taken a course from the Dalai Lama at the University of Virginia, she had me order a copy of Sharon Salzberg's tapes for Mittie for Christmas.

Bob Karlson and The Healing Temple

Bob Karlson was my department chair when I began teaching at George Mason in 1966, and introduced me to meditation in 1973. When he learned that Diana was ill, he invited us to visit him so he could help Diana with relaxation exercises, which we did. His home was only a few miles from Fairfax hospital where we went for surgery, radiation, and chemotherapy. Bob also taught

Diana a basic relaxation technique in which she focused on one part of the body at a time, starting with her feet and moving up her body, saying to herself, "I'm relaxing my feet, I'm relaxing my feet, my feet are relaxed." The parts of the body Bob included were as follows:

    Calves
    Thighs
    Buttocks
    Abdomen
    Lower back
    Stomach muscles
    Upper back
    Chest muscles
    Forearms
    Upper arms
    Shoulders
    Facial muscles
    My whole body

    I couldn't tell how much she used this technique, but I do know she enjoyed learning it.

    When Diana had a downturn in the spring of 1997, Bob visited a few times and brought with him Jack Kornfield's book, *A Path with Heart*. At the end of the chapter on healing, Kornfield has a guided meditation exercise (pp. 54–55). I modified it for Diana, and we used it regularly in her last year. I sat on my bed and said the following in a gentle, relaxed voice, pausing frequently. Again, this is my modified version of Kornfield's guided meditation.

> Relax your body, and for a moment, pay attention to your breath. Don't try to change your breath, just pay attention to it. Notice anything about it that is comfortable or uncomfortable. Also pay attention to your heart, and

notice if it feels contracted or soft and open. Take a minute to pay attention to it.

Imagine yourself in a beautiful healing temple, a place of great wisdom and love. Take as much time as you need to sense it, to feel it, to picture it in any way you wish. Imagine yourself sitting in the temple, this place of great wisdom, and begin to reflect on your own spiritual journey. Gradually, let yourself be aware of the wounds you carry that require healing in the course of your journey. Breathe softly, and feel whatever arises.

As you sit in this healing temple, a wonderful and wise being will gently approach you. When this being comes quite near you, you can sense who he or she is. This person will bow lightly and then come over and put a hand on a part of your body where you are deeply wounded. Let this person touch the part of your body that holds one of your sorrows. Let this person teach you the healing touch. If you like, imagine placing your own hand on your deepest wound, your place of sorrow or difficulty, touching it with your hand as if you yourself were that beautiful being. Know that no matter how many times you have resisted your sorrow, you can now open to it.

Let your attention become like the hand of this wonderful wise being. Touch this place with softness and tenderness. As you touch it, explore what is there. Is it warm or cool, is it hard and tight, or is it soft? Is it vibrating or moving, or is it still? Let your awareness be like the loving touch of the Buddha or the Goddess of Compassion, of Mother Mary or Jesus. Let yourself become aware of your feelings with a very loving and receptive heart. Let them be anything they need to be. Then very gently and softly, as if you were the Goddess of Compassion herself, touch it with pure sweetness. Open yourself to the pain. Let yourself sit peacefully, opening your heart to this pain.

Rest in this temple, allowing your healing and compassionate attention to move into every part of it. Stay as long as you wish. When you are ready to leave, imagine yourself bowing with gratitude. As you leave, remember this temple is inside you. You can always go there.

Diana was very peaceful after these guided meditations. I know that my goal was total and complete recovery, but I also know that the odds of that happening were slight. So if the tumor returned, at least her spirit would be healed, and that would be the most important part.

Diana frequently requested that I read Kornfield's book to her, and we made it through half the book before she died.

Rhiannon

On February 12, 1997, I got a reading from Rhiannon, a gorgeous, young, red-headed, Welsh psychic I had met around 1989. In previous readings, she had helped me make decisions that were in my best interest even though I didn't like admitting it at the time. Rhiannon used to visit Warrenton, but had moved further away, so this reading she conducted over the phone.

I asked her for a reading because I was afraid Diana was going to die—and not knowing the future was so frightening. I thought I could remedy with Rhiannon's help. I had called Rhiannon sometime around Diana's stay in the hospital or several weeks before the reading. I believe I told her that Diana had been diagnosed with brain cancer and that I was in some turmoil about her surviving the illness. The focus of the reading was Diana's death—in other words, Rhiannon confirmed the prognosis of the doctors. If Rhiannon were correct, therefore, I could shift my energies away from wondering whether she would die, to doing something about the time we had left. I told Diana countless times that my goal was to bring about a total and complete recovery—and until such time as it was evident that she was dying, all my efforts would be to get her back on her feet and back to as normal a life as possible. I considered both the prognosis of the doctors and the reading from Rhiannon as opinions from experts—but neither were fact until they happened.

I also asked for a reading because Rhiannon's perspective was much larger than mine, and included the spiritual dimension that I needed. I tend to think that all we have is this life, this world. Unlike some people who commune with spirits, I don't know what lies on the other side. I've read about it but have no experience with the after life.

Rhiannon scheduled the reading for February 12, at 10:00 in the morning. I know from other readings I received from Rhiannon, ones in which I was sitting across from her rather than listening to her over the phone, that she would begin by sitting for a moment and praying, asking God for guidance and for her powers be used to benefit mankind. Then she would be very quiet and wait for several moments, switching her mind so that she was not talking but listening. Then she would jot down in an almost illegible handwriting what she heard, read it aloud to me, discuss it and elaborate on it, allow time for me to ask questions, and, at the end, would give me the pages of writing she had taken down.

Because this was a reading she did over the phone, she had already written down what she heard, and, therefore began by reading it aloud to me. The following is what she read to me. Marisa and I put it into poetry format, but otherwise, it is as she wrote it.

> Be ye still and know that time runneth short
> unto the way of freedom and of peace
> for she who dwells with thee.
>
> Blessed be thy journey;
> blessed be the formation of thy way;
>   and yet as Death knocks upon thy door,
>   and the carriage awaits her enlightened soul,
>   still there lies sorrow and resistance in thy separation.

Finished Business

Yet within each grain of emotion thou would feel—
there lies peace beyond thine own mental understanding.

The comforter is with thee anointing both thy heads
and the way paved with precious jewels and rose petals
that fall about thy feet.

This is thy sacred time given unto each of thee
to move closer unto the garden of thine own blessed unity.
Time is not thine enemy.
It is thine healer and passageway
unto the whole of all that thou are
in glory of thy truth.

And where she shall walk,
thou too will follow in time passing.
Yet thy journey continues to unwind and meander a new song.
For this song at this here time
moves unto the mellowness and the depth of great compassion,
leading thee to drink from the great well of communion.
For even though one prepares to cross the veil,
there shall lie no separation in thine hearts and soul.
The song remains clear and fresh as the new day begun,
dear in thy spirit, Death robs thee not of thy treasure.

Take ye the days numbered
as dew drops falling upon thy face.
In beauty of arising with her—
steadfastly walking her gently to the gateway,
where along thy way,
the scenes of day-to-day life seem adorned with new insight
unto the great plight of her spirit.
And there at the gateway come many to receive her,
many to show her the wonder of flight.

Look not down upon the ground in fear,
for thy days shall be as sacred—as thy first breath taken unto life itself
and unto her cometh great joy and acceptance of her calling.
Her kin is watching and standing by
and even though thine heart is aching,
thy tears shall too set thee free
into the greater capacity of thy higher being.

Walk forwards with courage, my friend
for in but a twinkle of an eye
in the span of living left for thee in thy domain,
thou shalt too arise to meet her happy eyes
and thy quest shall ever continue
in the new melodies the future will form.

Thy days remaining whilst She flies
shall not be cold nor dark nor depraved of light,
for thou too shall receive wings to fly,
aware of her presence by thy side—
guiding, bestowing the wonder of her sight.

Follow onwards dear friend,
for thy moments are filled with illumination
and healing hands that come to soothe the pain
and keep thee safe from the fear of loss.

Thou art armed with light
and protected with understanding
that the dawn will soon rise
for fast moves the tide inwards towards thee all,
to carry what is of essence back unto the all good Creator of all.

And thy boat is weak, yet the sail is strong
as thou would carry her hither to the happy throng
awaiting to celebrate her crossing of the way,
saluting thee, her blessed one,
that still hath many a day to walk upon soil.

Bells are ringing
and her mother is singing—
rejoicing the birth of her incoming one.

Peace.

After she read this to me, she went over what she considered the key elements—that this was a sacred time for us, that there was great compassion between Diana and me, and that death wasn't robbing us of our relationship. She said that if you have no heavy karma, you can continue your life in the spirit world—and Diana had no heavy karma. She said the pathway or oneness of spirit Diana and I shared was just beginning and that we had many lifetimes to come. She said many were coming to greet Diana on the other side and that foremost among them were her mother.

Rhiannon saw the near future, between February and March of 1997, as a time of healing. She talked about our having the rest of this year (1997) during which Diana would have a renewal of strength and would feel more vibrant about life. She said Diana would die in the springtime (she did not say which Spring, and I did not think to ask) when the birds return to the south and the flowers are in bloom. She also said that I would be there when her spirit left her body and that I would somehow participate in her dying—like carrying a child over to her mother. She said we would have no unfinished business, and she would die peacefully.

She said that I, too, was receiving my "wings" and that the light from this experience is more than I could envision, and it would change my whole life. My journey with Diana would continue after her death and later after mine. After Diana died, I would still have many days left on this earth, but perhaps not as many as I thought. I would have access to her, and she would bless my continued journey in this world. She said Diana would see me but that I wouldn't see her. She saw my path merging with groups of people during the rest of 1997, perhaps spiritual groups. She said Diana would be there to guide me when I died.

I asked her about how our three children would deal with her illness and death. Rhiannon said that they would have time with her and that she would have time to speak and bestow her love on them. She said John would have the greatest sadness, yet there would be lots of compassion between them. She thought Diana might visit John first after she died. She saw sadness in Brendan yet a sense of freedom and a new path forming. She saw lots of healing and compassion between Diana and Marisa and had a strong feeling of birth around her. She thought Marisa would have a baby within two years and that Diana would have time with this child.

Rhiannon asked me to purify water and bless it in the sunlight, then give it to Diana and anoint her head with it to ease the pain. I was also to drink this water. (I poured filtered water into a glass, held it up to the sun light, blessed it, and gave it to Diana to drink. I also anointed her head with it and then drank it myself. I did this several times during the spring of 1997.)

I asked Rhiannon if I should tell Diana about this tape, and she advised me to wait a while because Diana knew she was not facing death just yet. I also asked her if I had anything to do with causing Diana's illness, and Rhiannon said these things are beyond our control, and there was no need to put such things on myself. She said the illness could have come from fear, from her mother, genetically from previous generations—only the Creator knew, and it was not necessary for us to know the cause.

Rhiannon saw a shift occurring on the 16th of February, but I couldn't verify that from my medical records or journal entries for 1997 or 1998. Perhaps it had something to do with her spiritual life. I really don't know.

My journal does contain this exchange that took place sometime in the middle of February 1997, prompted, I would guess, by the tape.

> Don: I love the spirit that's inside this body [pointing to her chest]. You're a good traveling companion. Do you think we've traveled together before in previous lives?
>
> Diana: No. You're too strange.
>
> Don: Do you think we'll travel together in subsequent lives?
>
> Diana: I hope so.
>
> Don: Me too.

Sister Donald and Frank Culley

Sister Donald Cocoran is a friend of Diana's cousin Virginia, and, through Virginia, learned about Diana's illness. Sister Donald visited once on August 13, 1997 and had previously sent us a copy of her book *Spiritual Sisters*, which she co-authored with Venerable Thubten Chodron. It is a book on interreligious dialogue, written by a Benedictine nun and a Buddhist nun, with an additional chapter containing a talk by His Holiness the Dalai Lama to Christian monks as well as an article by a Buddhist nun who visited an Anglican convent. The book was interesting for us because Diana and I had found our childhood Catholicism benefiting from exposure to Buddhist ideas. As I mentioned earlier, the year before she became ill, she read Sharon Salzberg's *Lovingkindness*, a book on the art of happiness by a Buddhist. I had been reading Buddhist texts since the early 1980's.

Sister Donald was born in Minnesota and has been a Benedictine nun for over 35 years. She also has a Ph.D. in theology from Fordham University, and, in 1979, helped found the Transfiguration Monastery in Windsor, New York.

When Sister Donald visited, Diana was weak. She was able to chat with Sister Donald, but was bedridden. The three of us chatted for about ten minutes, then Sister Donald asked Diana if she would like her to say a prayer for her. "I'd like that very much," Diana said. When Sister Donald placed her left hand on Diana's head and began to pray, Diana wept. She didn't cry or sob or whimper, she wept—the soft, gentle tears of one touched to the core. Sister Donald's words were spontaneous, asking Jesus to heal her. The touch, even though I could not feel it myself, looked powerful, calm, and reassuring.

When I walked Sister Donald downstairs to the door, she turned to me and asked me about Diana's prognosis. Then she said she would continue to pray for her.

It was hard to tell if the changes I saw in Diana's condition over the next few weeks were real or imagined, but I thought I saw improvement.

Our friend, Frank Culley spent about 15 years as a Trappist monk. He left the monastery and married a teacher I worked with for many years. Frank is a large man with hands you get lost in when you greet him. When he came to visit Diana, at about the same time as did Sister Donald, he was his usual quiet self. During his first of two visits, Diana was very weak and did not wake. Frank sat in the chair next to her bed, lowered his head, closed his eyes, and prayed silently for about ten minutes. Then he placed his large hand on her head, right where her tumor had been. I wondered how he knew where it was because I had not told him, and no scar was visible from the surgery. Perhaps it was coincidental. He left his hand on her head for about five minutes while he continued to pray.

Again, as with Sister Donald, I noticed improvement during the weeks after his visit.

I feel very fortunate and grateful that these two people visited Diana. I don't know what happened with her spirit, but I do know that I sensed a calmness and courage in them that they were able to transfer to her.

Faith of our Fathers—The CD

When we first heard "Faith of our Fathers: Classic Religious Anthems of Ireland" on a National Public Radio fund raiser, Diana cried, and as I held her head in my arms, I cried along with her. She asked me to order a copy. When it arrived, we played it numerous times, and I think it led to her reconciliation with the Catholic Church.

The music is sung and played with fervor. The voices of tenor, Frank Patterson, and soprano, Regina Nathan, are quintessential Irish Catholic, rising above the Irish Philharmonic Orchestra and Chorus. Diana cried often while listening to this CD, and mostly during "I'll Sing a Hymn to Mary" sung by child soprano Ros Ni Dhubhain. Dhubhain's voice is the voice of an innocent, ringing out with an utterly defenseless faith and trust. Not until writing this section did I make the connection between Diana's identifying herself as a mother and the motherhood of Mary in the hymn. As I mention elsewhere, the only wish Diana had was for her children to be happy.

Here are the words to the hymn:

I'll sing a Hymn to Mary,
The Mother of my God,
The Virgin of all virgins,
Of David's royal blood.
Oh! Teach me, holy Mary,
A loving song to frame,
When wicked men blaspheme thee,

To love and bless thy name
O Lily of the Valley
O Mystic Rose, what tree–
Or flower, e'en the fairest–
Is half so fair as thee?
Oh! Let me, though so lowly,
recite my mother's fame:
When wicked men blaspheme thee,
I'll love and bless thy name.

There is a purity to the refrain that is much like the philosophy of Sharon Salzberg's *Lovingkindness* and Diana's thoughts and actions in the last year of her life—return love for hate. There is some reason to believe it was influenced by the cancer, but I also think it is a result of Diana letting go. I saw her return to innocence—not innocence born of ignorance, but innocence born of experience. When life dealt her brain cancer, she returned to life with love and compassion for others.

Father Riley and Reconciliation with the Church

On Monday, September 29, 1997, while Julie was sitting with Diana while I went to yoga class, Julie and Diana talked about several things including the church. Julie asked her if she were interested in seeing a priest. Diana had been listening to "Faith of Our Fathers" for about a month and had received Sister Donald and her childhood friend Mary Jo in August. I believe she was thinking more and more about the church and what it had meant to her. Diana said, "No, yes, no, maybe." The next day, Julie, while out running her dogs at St. John's Catholic Church, saw Father Riley and said, "I have a friend who is interested in having a visit from a priest." We were moved that Julie referred to Diana as a friend and not a patient. Father Riley called and visited on Friday, October 3rd.

Father Riley was an elf of a man—or perhaps I should say imp of a man. He was short, quick, dark-haired, and dark-eyed Irish. Even though he was from Philadelphia, his voice sounded as if he recently left Ireland. I met him at the door and walked him up the stairs. Even though Diana had been regaining strength in September and October, she was still bedridden, and talked to Father Riley while lying on her back in bed. He held her hand.

I sat in the wing chair for the first 20 minutes or so while Father Riley and Diana talked. Father Riley was very direct, almost pushy, but kind and considerate. He said he had brought the Eucharist and wanted to know if she were interested in receiving it. He reiterated his offer throughout the conversation as if he were a salesman. Then Father Riley said, "So, what has kept you from the church?" Diana talked about the three things. She thought it was wrong that the Pope did not take a stand on the wrongness of the Vietnam War. She spoke of the My Lai massacre and the church's silence. I remember our going to mass at St. Leo's in Fairfax after the news of the massacre had broken, and the pastor of the church gave a long sermon on tithing. For about a year, we had been disappointed with the lack of spiritual content in the sermons at St. Leo's. Father Riley's response was that it was wrong of the church to do so, but quickly asked Diana if she had ever made a mistake and if she could find it in herself to forgive the church. "Thirty years was a long time to hold this against the church," he said.

Diana talked about the baptism of our children—about the liturgy that talks about their being born in mortal sin. I remember her turmoil in the late sixties when she said her babies were innocent—they were not in sin. She thought the church was wrong about original sin.

Diana also talked about the refusal of the church to admit women into the priesthood. Father Riley responded to her last two comments with traditional church doctrine without dismissing her views.

At the end, Father Riley asked her if she would like to make her confession.

She laughed and said it would take a long time. Father Riley said he didn't need to hear all the particulars, so he would go through the Ten Commandments. "If I do this," she said, "what am I obligating myself to?"

"When you're up to it, come back to church," Father Riley said. "Would you like to say your confession?"

"Yes," she said.

I turned off the monitor and went down stairs. About ten minutes later, Father Riley called down from the upstairs hallway to say that she was having a seizure. I ran up, held her, and talked to her until she calmed down. When she was ready to continue, I left, she finished her confession, and received communion.

I walked Father Riley to the door, then returned to the bedroom and asked Diana what she thought about returning to the church. "If I don't like it, I can leave again," she said, then laughed. I think she was a little overwhelmed by the reconciliation, but also glad she did it.

Bernie Reagan's Visits on Wednesdays

We had met Bernie and Peg Reagan shortly after we moved to Warrenton in 1975. We had attended a Marriage Encounter retreat in 1973, and even though we had our own Marriage Encounter group from our days in Farifax, we wanted to continue to meet people in Warrenton who also had a stake in working at their marriages. The Reagans held numerous meetings at their home, and we got to know them socially as well. Over the years, however, with the demands of commuting and rearing children, we lost contact with them. We saw them from time to time on the street and knew that Bernie had retired and become a deacon at St. John's.

Bernie would call earlier in the week and come with the Eucharist on Wednesday afternoons. Bernie is a shy, introspective man with a full head of white hair who came to the house in a dark suit and black overcoat that our black-and-white-haired cat loved to shed on. Bernie's job was to bring the Eucharist to Diana and visit the sick. Because he was also a friend, and because Diana enjoyed his visits, he would stay about an hour talking with her about family, the church, current events, and whatever else was on her mind. According to his own account, she drew him out, and their conversations were relaxed and friendly.

Outside/Inside
(After reading Zen Mind, Beginner's Mind)

The following is an undated entry from my journal during the year Diana was sick:

> People on the outside look on this experience romantically as if this is something wonderful or heroic. But on the inside, it is nothing special. It is folding laundry, cooking meals, giving Diana a bath and helping her to brush her teeth, holding her when she cries, listening to her words, giving her a bedpan, or changing her diapers throughout the night. I look on people who come to visit us as unusual; they look on us as unusual. We each are ordinary in our own worlds.
>
> In the beginning, I looked on this as unusual. I was helping someone to prepare to die, or I was helping someone survive a life threatening illness. The first time I talked to the health insurance people, the first time I walked Diana to the radiation table, it was special. I was doing something unusual. I was special; we were special. These things done day after day are no longer special. They are ordinary.
>
> The thoughts I had before Diana got sick were the same thoughts I have now. The struggles are the same, one being to do each thing with attention and love. The consequences are the same. When I feed Diana a spoon of

mixed fruit with love in the pace of the spooning, she feels loved. I never know when her last spoonful will be. Before Diana got sick, it was the same, and I never knew when my talking with her would be the last words she would hear from me. If I spoke with love, she felt loved.

So, whenever possible, I do things with love.

Novena

Diana was in touch with her cousin George Mason who also had had cancer. I dialed his number three or four times during the year and Diana talked to him for ten or fifteen minutes each time. He mentioned a novena that he had been saying to help himself recover from cancer, and when Diana asked for it, he sent it along.

According to the pamphlet that contained the novena, Anthony Claret was a Spanish priest who founded the Claretian Fathers in 1849. He was very sick twice during his own lifetime and had miraculous recoveries through the intercession of the Blessed Virgin Mary.

By the time we received the novena, Diana was blind, so she never had a chance to read it herself. Consequently, I read it for her, usually the last thing at night before going to sleep. She would say the three prayers at the end of the novena, then we would both say, "Amen."

I substituted the pronoun "we" for "I" because I was saying the novena along with and for Diana. In the section in parenthesis that asks you to mention the person afflicted with cancer or other serious ailment, I included Diana's name, and Diana asked me to include five other people who were also ill. It was typical of her to think of other people.

Novena to Saint Anthony M. Claret

In the name of the Father, and the Son, and the Holy Spirit. Amen.

Eternal and merciful God, in Your infinite bounty You have chosen Anthony Mary Claret to be a model and example for all mankind. We humbly ask You to bless us with his virtues and to grant us the graces that we need, especially those which we ask through his intercession in this novena. Hear his prayers, most merciful Lord, and kindly accept them in accordance with the tenderness of Your Sacred Heart. Amen.

Prayer to Saint Anthony Claret for the Cure of Cancer or Other Serious Ailments

Saint Anthony Claret, who during your life on earth were often a solace to the afflicted, and did love and tenderly compassionate the sick, intercede for us as you rejoice in the reward of your virtues. Cast a glance of pity on (here mention the person afflicted with cancer or other serious ailment) and grant our petition if such be the will of God. Make our troubles your own. Ask the Immaculate Heart of Mary to obtain by her powerful intercession the grace we yearn for so ardently, and a blessing that may strengthen us during life, assist us as the hour of death, and lead us on to a happy eternity. Amen.

Saint Anthony Claret, pray for us!

This was followed by one Our Father, one Hail Mary, and one Glory Be to the Father.

I could not tell how much Diana believed in the power of this novena. I do know that if I forgot to say it, she would remember. I have no way of judging the effect of our saying it. That it was something Diana wanted to do was sufficient reason to do it.

Chanting

In the last four months of her life, Diana would nap in the late afternoon, usually around 5:00. I looked down on her with a sickening sadness in my chest and with relief that she was getting rest. Sometimes, I would prepare dinner or return calls. If nothing were pressing, I would chant.

I slid my meditation cushion out from under my bed and positioned it between us. I slipped off my sandals, inserted a tape into the boom box, pushed the play button, and sat cross-legged in the half-lotus position on the cushion.

The tape was called "*The Gyuto Monks: Tibetan Tantric Choir.*" Mickey Hart, ethnomusicologist and drummer with the Grateful Dead, had produced both a special benefit concert of these Tibetan monks who were living in exile near Bombi-La, India, as well as the recording session that followed. Even though the chanting is spiritual (the tape insert says it is "prayer not performance"), I chanted to empty my chest of the sadness that built up over the day. The monks chanted an octave lower than I can, and each monk simultaneously sings a three-note chord. I tried to imitate them and but did not come close. Instead, I chanted an octave higher and in monotone, following their lead by raising one note at the end of the "refrains." The words were, to me, unrecognizable, so I used "*awe*" for the lower note, and "*oooh*" for the higher. I relaxed the back of my throat and let the sound vibrate through my head, throat, and chest.

Within a minute of my starting to chant, I could hear Diana's breathing deepen, which I interpreted she could hear both me and the tape. She never woke through the whole twenty-five minutes and seemed peaceful.

Usually, about five minutes into the chant, I would cry—always quietly so as not to disturb Diana, but sometimes hard, almost sobbing. Paying attention to her during the day was by now easy and joyful, but when I stepped back for a moment, I felt enormously sad. Ironically, I also missed her when she slept, even though she was inches away. I would cry for half a minute or so and return to the chanting, pushing out the vowels as loud and deep and hard as I could. For the first ten minutes, I felt as if I were forcing out the sound. After that, the chanting became easier, and just as powerful. I was going out of myself as well as moving beyond the garbage cans of emotion.

At the end of the tape, I felt much more peaceful. Proof of this would appear in the attention I subsequently gave Diana, or the hugs I gave people who visited in the evenings. In the months following her death, I have chanted regularly. It has helped the grieving, especially when my mind wanders onto something associated with Diana as I am chanting.

Transcending through Being in the Moment

I know a man whose life never quite equalled the glory of high school football. He spoke of it frequently and, if given the chance, would have relived it. I know a woman whose constant expression is, "Some day…" He's escaping into the past, she into the future.

I've spent my fair share of running away from the present and escaping into imagination. I've even had my share of transcending the present through prayer and things spiritual.

Working with Diana didn't allow for escaping. Not only did I have to pay attention to the present so that I wouldn't make mistakes, I also was drawn into the present by her groundedness in it. And I saw others drawn into it as well.

What I learned from hours and hours of paying attention to the present is that there is a transcendence that goes through the present, through being in the moment. The swirl of emotions and reasoning ceased when I gave my full attention to feeding her a spoonful of apple sauce, washing her face, or exercising her arm.

I used an exercise I teach my writing students. When a thought came along, I labeled it, watched it for a moment, and let it go. Most of my thoughts fit into two categories—fear and desire. Another way I looked at it was that one group of thoughts pushed me back and another pulled me forward. To be free, I let go of both and stood erect, leaning neither direction. At those moments, I moved through the present to the infinite—a place where the sequence of nows stopped and there was only now. I watched my hand holding the spoon move to her mouth, watched the spoon touch her lower lip, watched her mouth open, and watched the applesauce slide in. At such moments, I was neither reluctant to feed her nor eager to feed her. I just fed her.

Even when weak and blind, Diana sensed such moments. She called them love, and she felt very well taken care of. I thought of them as paying attention, and I loved her when I did.

Visiting Relatives as Entities

On January 29, 1997, Diana was in the hospital because she was having trouble regulating her medications. At around 3:00 in the morning, she called me over to her bed and said, "Grandma May is here," she said. Grandma May died in 1975.

"Do you see her or have a sense of her being here?"

"She's here, and so is Aunt Jess, and my mother."

I had read and heard of the dead relatives of dying people coming to see them. I didn't think Diana was sick enough to die, so I was surprised at the visits.

This was also the time when she began to have hallucinations. I had a sense that her relatives visiting were different from the hallucinations, but I wasn't sure why. When I looked around the room, I did not see anything unusual, and I did not feel cold spots, nothing moved, and my hair didn't stand on end. Nevertheless, I believed that her relatives were there.

A few days later when they were still there, I asked Diana, "What are they doing here?"

"Setting things in order."

"Setting things in order?"

"Setting things straight," she said.

When Diana returned home, the relatives followed, and were in her room for about a month. When Mittie, from Hospice, first came into Diana's room, she said she sensed that there were spirits there.

As far as I can tell, the spirits left in February 1997, after we got a routine in place to take care of Diana. They returned about a month before she died and left for good at her death. I never saw or sensed them, but that Diana did was good enough for me. I think she felt comforted by their presence, and enjoyed their coming to take care of things.

Death

The Decline

Looking through the records, the first hint of Diana's decline can be seen at the end of December 1997, in Julie's physical therapy notes: "decreased shoulder range of motion." On December 29th, Diana told Julie that she felt some tingling in her left fingers, and they intermittently felt like being stuck by pins. Looking back now, I can see this was a result of the tumor. At the time, however, we were elated at her progress, and the hope that it would continue clouded our seeing tingling as anything more than a passing problem.

On January 8th, 1998, Julie noticed that Diana needed considerable verbal cues for turning around and tended to forget where her left arm was when she was working on the parallel bars. Also during that visit to the hospital, Diana became tired and had to sit down.

By January 14th, Diana needed constant reminders to move her left arm forward while working with Julie on the parallel bars, and tended to lean forward and to the left.

The following is the progress of her decline.

January 16, 1998 — Diana was weak at the pool and leaned to the left the more tired she became. She also was unable to hold on to the left dumbbell and lost it more than 20 times. When she tried to walk up the stairs to get out of the pool, her legs buckled, and she had to use the chair lift.

January 17, 1998 — Diana slept a lot.

January 19, 1998 — Diana walked down and up the stairs in the house and walked down the stairs in the pool but not up. She lost the left dumbbell more than 30 times in the pool, but seemed to have better balance.

January 21, 1998 — At home, Carol walked Diana to the bathroom. Diana had enough strength to get there, but when she tried to stand up from the commode, she couldn't. "You tell me what is the best position to get you up," Carol told her. Carol was thinking that she might have to call some of her friends at the rescue squad to help get Diana back to bed. Diana said, "Donald just lifts me up." Carol, being considerably shorter, didn't have that option. They tried different positions, and finally Diana managed to stand. When Carol offered the walker, Diana said, "I don't need it."

"Humor me," Carol said. Diana shuffled back to the bed, listing to the left.

January 27, 1998 — Diana walked down the stairs at home, then folded. She used the chair lift to enter and exit the pool. She had great difficulty with the shower after the pool and with getting dressed, and was too weak to stand and pivot safely. I remember being quite alarmed at her weakness in the shower, and there were moments I feared she might collapse on the floor, wet and naked. I also remember thinking the therapists in the pool area had heard me raise my voice at Diana when she wasn't able to respond. It was, as the expression goes, a bad scene.

January 29, 1998 Diana went to the hospital for physical therapy, but she was weak. Julie wrote in the chart, "The patient reports she is doing well. The patient's husband reports she has been extremely fatigued and tired." This is typical Diana—saying she is fine even when she is not. Diana began therapy at the hospital by walking about eight feet holding on to the parallel bars, and then rested for five minutes. Then she walked sideways for three steps and had to sit down. Julie and Barbara then re-evaluated Diana's condition and noticed that she was unable to move her arm at all well, so they gave her a moist hot pack for 25 minutes and soft tissue massage to her back and left arm for another ten minutes. This was the last day she was to leave the house.

January 30, 1998 Diana was too weak for the pool.

February 2, 1998 Diana had a bad seizure that included her left arm shaking. She also had a bowel movement in her pants.

February 3, 1998   Diana was too weak for the pool. She had a bad headache and had trouble standing. We had a system for determining the severity of the headaches. I would ask her to give me a read on a scale of one to ten. On this day it was a 3 so I gave her Ibuprofen that gave her relief.

February 6, 1998   Diana had a severe headache and was incontinent most of the day. She almost seized when I changed the sheets. Some of the headaches became an eight, then a nine, and finally they were hitting a ten, even once a twelve. With Dr. Maybach's approval, I gave Diana Tylenol with Codeine. I hated putting her back on this because, even though it relieved her headaches, it also produced constipation and sleepiness.

February 8, 1998   Diana projectile vomited once today. Everything she had eaten she spewed out of her mouth and nose.

February 9, 1998   I came home from teaching around 11:00 p.m. Diana seemed fine. Suddenly, at 12:30 a.m., she projectile vomited all over the bed and sheets. I managed to get her and the bed cleaned up, changed the sheets and her pajamas, gave her a sponge bath, washed her hair with a washcloth, and settled her down when she vomited again, almost identically to the first. I again cleaned her up, changed pajamas and sheets, and this time placed a sheet around her chest. When she seemed comfortable, around 1:30 a.m., I gathered up the sheets and clothes and carried them downstairs. Just as I was stuffing them into the washing machine, I could hear her over the monitor throw up again. I raced up stairs and felt so sorry for her. The vomit was everywhere, and her eyes were watering. After I cleaned her up this time, she fell asleep. The next morning, I called John and Dr. Maybach, and Dr. Maybach prescribed Phenergan suppositories to control the vomiting. Our best guess was that the tumor had reached a part of her brain that triggers vomiting.

February 25, 1998   Diana vomited but today it was not projectile vomiting. After talking to John, I checked her mouth, and his guess was right—Diana was not swallowing her meds. I crushed her meds with a mortar as I had a year earlier and mixed meds with applesauce that she swallowed without difficulty.

March 12, 1998   Diana seemed to urinate less, and I thought she might have a urinary tract infection, so I requested a Cipro prescription from Dr. Maybach. She began urinating regularly on the 15th and had no trouble with it afterward.

March 19, 1998   Diana had trouble chewing and swallowing, so I returned to a diet of mixed fruit and whatever else I could get into her. At around this time, she was incontinent, yet rather than place her back in diapers, which would be a clear sign she were regressing, I chose to keep her in pajamas. It was very little extra work changing the pajama bottoms and chucks, and it made her more comfortable. When I told Mittie, she thought it was the right decision.

From here on, Diana slept more and lost the strength she had worked so hard to gain back the year before. Her left side became less mobile, and then as the tumor progressed, she also lost mobility in her right side.

On March 19, 1998, I sent an e-mail note to a student who asked about Diana: "Diana is very weak but comfortable. We're pretty sure the tumor has spread to her left hemisphere. Her speech and right side of her body barely function."

The tumor had grown back in the right hemisphere of her brain and, in the last month of her life, crossed into the left just as the hospice volunteer had predicted.

Approaching Death

In the first week of March 1998, I knew Diana was considerably weaker, and I began to prepare her for death. The following is what I told her, with my notes resting on the head of the bed and my right hand stroking her forehead and hair. I wanted my hands and the tone of my voice to reassure her that everything would be OK.

"Sweetie, you've been sleeping a lot lately, and you've been eating less and drinking less. Do you know what is happening to you?"

"What?"

"I think you're beginning to make your transition. You're beginning to move into the spirit world."

"That's not my specialty," she said. We laughed.

"I'll be talking to you from time to time, telling you the same things over and over. You'll be able to hear me, and I want you to interrupt me whenever you have something to say. Do you understand this so far?"

"Yes."

"I don't know what happens when we die, but from what I've read, and from what some people say, this is what I think will happen.

"You've completed things on this side. You've been a wonderful wife, and mother, and now grandmother. So you have nothing left to do—you're leaving nothing undone.

"When we die, I think the spirit leaves through the head of the body and stays in the room for a short while. I don't know the exact length of time. Maybe it varies from person to person, but you'll be able to see us standing here—you'll probably see us crying. At that point, because you'll no longer have this body with you, you won't feel any pain. You'll watch us but you won't feel any discomfort. You'll know that we're OK—even though we're crying—and that you'll be free to continue on your journey.

"From what I've read, I think you'll be drawn to some kind of light—some people call it a tunnel with a bright white light at the end. I think that's where you'll meet people like your grandmother and your mom, and probably your dad and Aunt Jess and your other relatives who are on the other side.

"Somewhere around this time, you may see things that you are fond of, or things you are frightened of, and I think these things are just projections of your consciousness. All you need to do at this point is to realize that they are your projections, identify them as such, and let them go. I think it is something like your life passing before you. They're nothing to be worried about—so just know that they're coming from your consciousness, and you can let go of them.

"I also understand that when you get to the spirit world, you may be traveling from place to place—I don't know what these places are—but you'll also be able to come back and visit us from time to time, especially when we need you.

"This is all I know at this time. I'll be telling you the same things again several times so that you'll understand and have a chance to ask me questions."

I said the same thing to her a second time the next day, and at the point where she had previously said, "That's not my specialty," she said, "That's not good, is it?"

"No, it's not," I replied. I think she understood that she really was getting weaker and would be dying in the near future.

On the third day, I repeated the same things to her, and this time she said, "I hope you'll be here."

"I'll be here," I said.

Preparations and The Tibetan Book of the Dead

I first heard of *The Tibetan Book of the Dead* when I read Walt Anderson's *Open Secrets: A Western Guide to Tibetan Buddhism* in the early 1980's. At the time, I had no idea I would ever be in a position to help someone, much less my wife, die. I read it because so many Buddhist writers referred to it. After Diana became ill, I also ran across several references to it in the literature on death.

According to Anderson, it is Tibetan custom to read *The Tibetan Book of the Dead* aloud in the house of the dying. "It is a set of instructions to the deceased about how to deal with the experiences encountered immediately after death in the bardos, or planes of existence, beyond ordinary life," (Anderson 1980, p. 150). The book describes opportunities for enlightenment that will free people from the cycle of death and rebirth. If the dying do not become enlightened, they are reborn.

According to *The Tibetan Book of the Dead*, the first opportunity for enlightenment is at the time of death and comes in the form of a clear light, which is a manifestation of the person's own consciousness. "If the deceased recognizes this light as the source of his or her own consciousness and identifies with it, liberation is achieved," (Anderson, 1980, p. 151). If the person misses this opportunity, a second opportunity follows, when he or she sees peaceful deities; if these opportunities are missed, a third opportunity arrives in the form of wrathful deities. How does this work? According to Anderson, "If the consciousness can recognize them [the white light, the peaceful and wrathful deities] as its own creations and thus become one with them, it has transcended the subject—object dichotomy that keeps it in its state of fearful confusion."

This thinking is an extension of the practice of meditation in which people learn to explore the subconscious and recognize its projections as their own creations—and then own them (Anderson 1980, p. 153. In other words, you free yourself from your own projections by facing them, by becoming one with them.

Carl Jung saw *The Tibetan Book of the Dead* as a map of the unconscious and the bardo experience as a form of therapy, a "penetration into the ground-layers of consciousness" similar to that undertaken in psychoanalysis, (Anderson, 1980, p. 156). To understand the book, Jung suggested reading it backwards, from the visions of wrathful deities to visions of peaceful deities and finally ending with the white light. This progression makes a great deal of sense to me when I think of using it as a guide for meditation. When I began meditating, I found myself facing my "wrathful deities" or menacing projections—including my fear of the devil. I vividly remember one meditation in which I was terrified that the devil was walking up the stairs to seize me. When I think of this book being read to a dying person, however, I would read it as it was written because, as far as I can tell, it follows the progression of death.

Jung also saw the interaction with the attending lama to be a form of psychotherapy—perhaps a last opportunity to put one's house in order. The Tibetan spiritual leader Chogyam Trungpa in his commentary to *The Tibetan Book of the Dead*, says such talk "presents tremendously rich inspiration to the dead person," and advises us to tell the dying person, "It [death] is actually happening, but we are your friends, therefore we are watching your death. We know that you are dying and you know that you are dying, we are really meeting together at this point," (Trungpa, 1975, p. 27). Simply put, having a friend or loved one hold your hand and talk you through your last moments can be very comforting.

During the year Diana was ill, I read this book several times, and briefly discussed it with her, more to let her know what I was doing than to instruct her on dying. Only when it was clear that she was dying did I use it as a basis for talking to her about death.

The Day Diana Died

At 2:00 a.m. on March 30, 1998, Diana's breathing became rapid. She seemed comfortable, and because I had no idea what was causing it, I was not alarmed. I turned her every two hours, and continued to check on her.

That morning, however, I was unable to get meds into her and knew things were not good. Sandy, the house cleaner, came at 9:00 a.m. and I had still not been able to get meds into Diana. When Carol came at 11:00 A.M., she said Diana was in shock. I didn't think death was imminent, so I drove to school to cancel class and collect papers. On the way, I called Brendan and told him that Diana had taken a turn for the worse. He called Marisa and John.

By 6:00 p.m., neither Carol nor I had been able to get meds into Diana. She breathed rapidly with her mouth open, and I knew instinctively that this kind of hard breathing could not go on indefinitely.

Brendan, Tracy, Nicholas, Diana, Glen, and Madeleine arrived in the early evening, along with Glen's parents, Jo and Bill Faunce. I knew we needed to get in touch with Dr. Maybach, and, through Julie, was able to reach him. He came over around

8:45. The room was oddly festive, despite Diana's condition. The children and grandchildren were in the room along with the mild chaos that accompanies small children. Dr. Maybach sat in the wing chair and discussed our options: to have her taken to the hospital; to insert a tube down her throat so that we could feed her the meds; or use an I.V. to give her liquids. I stood at the foot of the bed and told him I didn't want her taken to the hospital. When he mentioned the tube down her throat, Diana groaned disapproval. It was the first sign she had given us all day that she was conscious. Clearly, I was in favor of making her comfortable, but not prolonging her life.

Carol, who was standing beside the bed, wanted Dr. Maybach to examine her. She said Diana's pulse was 158 and her respiration rate was 158. She had been running a temperature slightly under 103 degrees Fahrenheit all day. Dr. Maybach walked over to the bed, checked her pulse and heart, then returned to the wing chair. He said she had one to three days to live. At that moment, Diana opened her eyes and looked right at me. I said, "We have eyes," and was delighted to see her respond. Things at this point were moving quickly. I was aware that she had heard our conversation. Her opening her eyes told me she knew her time was limited.

Around 9:20 p.m., Dr. Maybach rose to leave, so I walked him downstairs and thanked him for coming. When I returned to the room, Diana's breathing had changed. Tracy was standing beside her and said, "She's having sleep apnea." Only minutes before, she had slowed her breathing, waiting 10-15 seconds between breaths. Tracy said, "I think she's doing the apnea thing again. At first I thought so, too, but the breathing weakened. "That doesn't sound right," I said and traded places with her beside the bed. I looked closely at Diana and said, "She's dying." I looked up at Carol, who stood across the bed from me, for confirmation, although I didn't really need any. Carol was not able to find a pulse with the stethoscope and blood pressure cuff. She nodded her head and began to cry. Marisa stood beside me, sobbing. Brendan cried openly.

Death

Diana Elizabeth Batch Gallehr died at 9:30 p.m., Monday, March 30, 1998. She died because her heart gave out. She died because she had brain cancer. She died because she heard Dr. Maybach say around 9:15 that she had one to three days. She died because she heard us rule out options that would unnecessarily prolong her life.

She died with Marisa, Brendan, Carol, and me at her bedside, telling her we loved her. John had been on the phone with us throughout the day and passed along his, "Tell mommy I love her."

"You're the best mommy," Marisa said.

"Yes," said Brendan.

"I love you," we said.

I stroked her hair, moving my fingers and hand back across her head. It was a gesture I had used countless times in the past two months, and I knew she liked it. It was also comforting for me, this stroking her head and passing her hair between my fingers, over, and over, and over. Subliminally, I thought, "*If I continue to stroke, she will not die.*"

I kept my eyes on her neck, watching her pulse. I considered repeating the advice I had given her weeks earlier about how to let go when dying, but figured we had talked about it enough that she could handle it on her own. It was more important to tell her I loved her, to stroke her hair, to let her know we were there. Her last breath came and went. The pulse in her neck stopped. We waited and cried and told her we loved her. She just stopped. That's all—she just stopped.

"I love you, Daddy," I heard Marisa say. We hugged each other. I hugged Brendan.

I didn't want to stop running my fingers through her hair. Her mouth was open. Her eyes closed. Even though her skin had lost its elasticity because she had been in shock for the past 20 hours, breathing like a runner, it was still beautiful. The skin around her mouth and chin had turned yellow about ten minutes before she died, but the rest of her body looked healthy.

We stayed in the room, crying, talking, and numb.

After a few minutes, I called John. He had been on the verge of flying to Warrenton several times during the day, but both of us thought Diana had at least a week left—maybe two. I told him, "Mommy just died." I could hear him cry. I so wished he had been here with us.

I called Julie and Dr. Maybach. Then I called the funeral home.

We stayed in the room, talking, crying, and even laughing at times. I continued to straighten up the room, to fold towels, to put things away. It was what I did. I had been doing the same thing, sometimes 24 hours a day, for over a year.

After Death

Taking out the Clothes

Marisa and I did the clothes about two weeks after she died. I had already emptied her dresser. I threw out her underwear, nightgowns, and pajamas—too personal to give to charity. I bagged her socks and belts. I had organized her jewelry one evening with her while she was alive because we were looking for a few pieces that she wanted to give away. She had wheeled into the master bedroom, then transferred to one of the wing chairs. I had described each piece and put them in small boxes. I had put necklaces in one area, rings and pins in another. I now wish I had labeled each piece because I don't remember the origin of many of these pieces—rings and broaches in particular. A valuable piece of family history lost—a continuity broken.

I had gone through her clothes while she was alive—making sure I knew where everything was so that when she asked for it I could find it. There were only a few pieces I had been unable to find, including a white sweater which she asked for several times and which I later found in the attic. I regret not having found it while she was alive.

She had a rack of blouses, mostly white, in the blue room. Her coats, dresses, and suits were in the wardrobe in the green room, and her slacks, shoes and sweaters were in the hall wardrobe. Marisa and I brought them into the green room, placed them on one bed, and then Marisa decided which ones she wanted to keep for herself and which she wanted to give to charity. I had several large boxes on hand including a few boxes from Hospice that had contained chucks and diapers.

I don't think I could have sorted the clothes by myself. I needed Marisa there to bring in a sense of the public nature of this act. Diana's clothes did not have a distinctive smell or texture, but each piece did bring back a memory, such as her Pendleton gray overcoat in which she looked so elegant, her shoes that had molded to her feet, a sweater I had given to her at Christmas, and a green sweater Sandy had given to her during radiation.

As we were sorting through her clothes, it struck me as it had several times during our marriage that she wore simple clothes, good clothes, and elegant clothes. Nothing very complicated or splashy. This was an essential wardrobe. They said as much by what wasn't included as by what was.

I was sad because I loved her elegant simplicity. She seemed to sift out the flotsam before presenting herself. No angst, no discussion. Essential beauty. Lasting beauty.

I carried boxes to Marisa's car that were to go with her, and boxes to the van which were to go to the Ladies Auxiliary of Fauquier Hospital. An armful of long dresses and coats were still on hangers. I slipped my left thumb beneath the hooks and draped the clothes over my right arm, and I was fine until I walked out the front door. The clothes were heavy, and at that moment, I felt as if I were carrying Diana out of the house, over the very threshold I had carried her 23 years earlier.

I was enormously sad at that moment, and writing about it makes me cry and brings back that sadness. You never think when carrying your "bride" over the threshold that you may some day reverse the direction. The threshold is just a piece of wood, but it symbolizes the division between the public world and the private. Outside is our house; inside is our home. Outside is where we "prepare a face to meet the faces that we meet", and inside is where we show our insides, where we grow up—fighting, challenging, hating, and loving—and now, where we die.

There was a finality to carrying out her clothes that surpassed the funeral, and even the burial. She would now and forever live somewhere else, and this house is where she would visit. In the last year of her life, I loved her to pieces, and no matter where I live or who I live with, a part of me will always miss her.

Hospice Support

I was surprised when several weeks after the funeral, I received a call from Joy LeBaron, Director of Hospice Support of Fauquier County. I had pretty much expected hospice to disappear from my life after Diana died. Joy was calling to see how I was doing—and just as she did before Diana died, she listened with great understanding and compassion.

Hospice has a bereavement support group that I have not attended for several reasons. I think my three children and close friends constitute, for me, a support group that helps me to grieve whenever I need to. They are as close as the phone. If I did not have them, however, I would be very involved in the bereavement group because I know I couldn't grieve alone.

Mittie would say, "I'll see you next week," when she left on Wednesdays—except the Wednesday before Diana died. Mittie knew.

I also saw Mittie several times when I dropped off bread at the Hospice office. Because Diana was with hospice for over a year when the average time for hospice patients is one month, the volunteers knew us very well. When Mittie came to take care of her during the last month of her life, she teared up when I briefed her about Diana's decline. Mittie and Diana had become friends. As Mittie said, "You couldn't help but fall in love with Diana."

Joy also called me regularly after Diana's death to check up on me. I learned later that hospice keeps in touch with the surviving member for 13 months in order to help them get past the first anniversary.

Helping People Grieve

Diana and I were given three extraordinary children, and we managed, somehow, not to damage them. They grew up to be bright, beautiful, wonderful people. Helping them to grieve was my first priority after Diana died.

I remember when Diana's mother died in 1984. We were at the wake, and it was at the time when I was still learning to deal with emotion. I felt very sad but hadn't cried. I was fighting crying openly and hung out at the rear of the room where her body lay in the casket. Our three children were with me as Diana went to the front and mingled with her brothers, father, and other relatives and friends. I felt a knot in my stomach, and so did Marisa. I knew it was from not crying when I needed to, but I didn't know what to do about it. A few minutes later, Diana came to the back of the room and led us up to the casket. She brought the children right up to it and talked lovingly about their grandmother. The children broke down and cried. A short while later, I did, too. If Diana had not eased us into crying and grieving, it would have been much more difficult for us. I don't know how she knew to do it, and I admire her for the courage, wisdom, and gentle grace it took to guide us through.

I remembered this after she died. Brendan and Marisa had already cried, openly and fully, as Diana died. John, who did not see her body until the wake, cried when I called him with news of her death, and also cried at the funeral home. All of us cried when we needed to thereafter. We also talked about Diana frequently, especially when the memory of her was particularly strong. Brendan, for example, told us of the time Diana had bought him a present in the middle of summer because his birthday was in

February while the others had birthdays in July and August. She wanted him to have a present during the summer, too.

We called each other every day, and frequently, I called Marisa only to find she was on the other line talking to John or Brendan. One night, I called Marisa who, I discovered, was talking to Tracy while Brendan was on his car phone talking to John. "The whole family in on the phone to each other," she said. It was a wondrous experience.

I also made sure I called people who were close to Diana—friends, relatives, and those who took care of her—to see if they are OK, to give them a chance to talk about her, to help them to heal.

My father died when I was 23, and I was very angry at him. It took me seven years of dreams to work through that anger. During one dream, I swung out at him. I woke when my hand hit the headboard, cracking it. Luckily, I missed Diana. In another dream, I shot at him with a pistol—I don't remember any shots hitting him. At the end of seven years, I dreamed of embracing him, and the dreams stopped. My mother died when I was 22, and I rarely dreamed of her. She was an emotionally absent person, and I had trouble finding her to grieve for. I cried for her in Diana's arms five days after her funeral, but cried for her after that only when I was purposely grieving her out of my system so that I wouldn't be acting out old business. I think it took me much longer than seven years to let her go, and I have no recollection of a specific event when I had finished. I just know that I by the time I was in my 40's, I had finished. She joined my father as a memory and not an unaware force that directed my actions.

It took me two years to finish grieving for Diana. I think I had been grieving for her since the onset of her illness, and especially since late January, 1997, when it was clear to me she was going to die from this cancer. I cried all but a few days during her last year and a half and virtually every day for over a year after her death. After she died, I wrote about her nearly every day for about six months, and each time, I cried. After about a year, I cried less and less, and by the second year, I had finished. I'm sure that is exactly what Diana would have wanted me to do.

Flowers

When friends and relatives asked if they should send flowers or a donation to Hospice, I told them that Diana loved flowers. I have no idea if she saw them, but we did, and they were beautiful.

Much has been written about the American way of death—about how we spend inordinate amounts of money on funerals and graves. Some cultures reverse the process, spending a great amount of time with the dying person, then treat the corpse as a slab of meat. Some cultures actually throw the body to the dogs.

I don't like either extreme. I know in my head that Diana left her body when she died, that she had no more use for it, but I knew her only in her body, and after her spirit left, it was all I had. I wanted to have her body around as long as I could—at least until I got used to the idea that she was dead and that her spirit was elsewhere.

When the funeral was over, we took most of the flowers back to the house that made the house look beautiful. When people left, gradually over the next few days, the flowers remained and gave me a connection to her that I needed.

Since then, people have sent flowers—to us rather than to her—and they have been visible reminders that they love us. The great benefit of calls is an opportunity to help people grieve.

Aftershocks

If death is an earthquake, the unexpected reminders of it are like aftershocks. They come while your mind is focused on something else and can rattle you to the core.

Memories are stored in many parts of the brain, and only when those parts are accessed do the memories come rushing out. Some memories are stored with sensory memory—sights, smells, and sounds. Music in particular can take me unaware. Other memories are stored with old thoughts, while some are stored with plans for the future. The following are a few of the many aftershocks I experienced since her death.

I was editing slides I had taken from a trip to Germany the summer before Diana's illness. I selected slides I wanted to show at a photography class I was taking and needed to place them in a slide tray I could take to class. In the tray were slides I had taken about five years ago of a tractor, a girl in a hat, a drainage pipe, the bark of a tree—and in the middle of them a slide I never knew I had—of Diana with her arms around Marisa who was about 10. Diana looked so young and beautiful, so happy.

One day, I was doing yoga exercises on the rug in the room Diana died in. I had little trouble walking in and out of that room since she died, even taking photos of the room. But as I lay on the rug and raised my head, I saw the floor that I had wiped with a wet cloth every morning of her illness. The floor was now clean and didn't need wiping.

I bought a rosemary plant for the herb garden. Before planting it, I cut a sprig to make rosemary bread. One was not enough, so I returned to cut a second. A few minutes later, I discovered I needed a third. I had to stop. I could not kill this rosemary plant. I had had enough of death.

I found myself wanting to buy a hand gun. This desire came and went for months. I asked myself where this desire came from. Finally, I knew. I was angry at death. I wanted to blast away at vegetables like zucchini and acorn squash. The whole thing was weird.

I can't see any way to prevent or prepare for aftershocks. It is part of the ongoing work of grieving, of daily working on the business of facing a loss, of talking about it, of crying over it. I now expect aftershocks to continue as long as I have unexplored memories.

Crying

I cried in the shower as I relaxed, letting go of the grief just below the surface. I cried while chanting. I cried while exercising. I cried while doing yard work.

Crying during movement seemed to work best for me, movement where I could get the grief up and out. Sometimes, I sobbed, and my whole body seemed to tense and shake as if every cell hurt. Sometimes, I cried quietly, without tears, without sound.

It was no big deal. If I hadn't cried, however, I would have become tight, bottled up, and frozen in time.

I didn't always cry. I think I cried as a baby and a youngster, but I didn't much growing up. My father didn't cry. My mother didn't cry unless she was angry. When I was eleven, I was praised as a man for not crying when I was mauled by a dog. It had nothing to do with courage—I had forgotten how.

I cried once when I was sixteen in a football game when the tackle across from me dislocated my jaw with a quick right. I cried when my mother died. I was 23. I didn't cry again until I was 37, and then I asked a friend how it was done. She said, you feel this hard ball in your gut, and you bounce it around and get it to come up your throat and out of your mouth. I tried and tried, but I couldn't fee the hard ball. I knew it was there—I just couldn't feel it. I practiced. Eventually, I found it, and moved it, and over the years, I learned to cry.

Diana cried very little, but she knew how. She cried when she was frustrated, when she lost her mom and later her dad, when she saw her leg after it had been in a cast, when I was cruel to her, when the kids left the nest. By then, we both knew how to cry, and we could fill a basket with tissues if the occasion warranted. And in her last year, she sobbed at the thought of her dying and leaving the kids without a mother.

I suppose there are lots of things to be said in favor of crying, but the one I favor is that it means you aren't running away from sadness—either because you can't or because you choose to stay.

In the long run, it is much easier to cry as the grief arises than to avoid it or stuff it back down. Grief will only grow under such conditions. It takes courage to stand and watch that enormous sadness move about inside of us.

As far as I can tell, you don't cry after you die. I think you require a body for that. Grieving and crying seem synonymous, and those of us with bodies and limited perspectives need to do both.

Receiving Condolences

The condolence I like best is, "I'm sorry." I like knowing that my grief is significant enough to make others sad. It's that simple.

Another condolence I like is a Diana story. I miss her and stories about her bring her back to me if only for a few moments.

I like to talk to people who know how to listen. My children and closest friends are listeners. They know the pacing and rhythm of listening, the use of sounds to let me know they're still involved in the conversation, and the pause to think through a response. They feel comfortable asking real questions—that is, questions based in genuine curiosity, such as, "Do you feel lonely?" or "Are there times of the day that are worse for you than others?"

I tend to save crying for periods when I'm alone, but it is very helpful when people are empathetic enough that I can cry with them if I so choose.

People who have lost someone close to them often know from experience how to respond—and frequently, there is a quietness about them that comes from knowing the enormity of the grief. They are comfortable with talking or not talking about death.

Many people, however, have not had someone close to them die, and they are as awkward as I used to be. For the two or three moments they are talking with me, I can help them to understand a little about death and what it is like to live in its wake.

Some people have said, "Diana's in a better place now." It doesn't make sense to me to compare this place to any other. I believe we can do things in this world that we can't do in the next, and vice versa. Both have a purpose in the large scheme of things, and I don't believe she died to get to a better place.

Other people say, "It must be a relief to know she is no longer suffering." I think suffering is caused by our running after desires or running away from fears and both activities are worth avoiding. Diana suffered very little because she lived mostly in the present during the last year of her life. She did, however, live in pain because she had cancer. I don't think her pain was purposeless—in fact, if anything, she transformed the pain into an opportunity to reach out to people. And as much as I hated to see her in pain, and even though I did everything in my power to alleviate it, because of it, she was able to do things she was never able to do before.

One person told me that this is all part of God's plan, that God knew what he was doing in letting her get cancer, and that God never gives us more than we can handle. I know enough not to take such comments literally. I believe there to be people who have been talked to by God, but haven't met them. The people I've met are trying to understand life and death just as I am, and this is their way of coming to terms with it, of making sense of things. They mean well, and because they do, I find it easy to be compassionate and understanding of their desire to console me. The truth for me, however, is that I don't know what role God played in Diana's cancer. I have no evidence that he intervened in the natural flow of events to cause her cancer. And I think you can manipulate your perspective on any life to prove that God doesn't give you more than you can handle.

A number of people have said, "You were very fortunate to have had this time together." I like this comment because I agree. We were able to bring love back into our marriage, to meet our grandchildren in this life, and time to prepare for death.

There are moments when my grief has been so strong that I don't want the distance that any condolence describes. I just want someone to hold me.

I needed about a year to complete the major part of my grieving for Diana. I grieved every day—sometimes crying openly, long, and hard. Other days, I sat down beside my sadness and let it talk. I tried not to cling to it or avoid it. I felt appreciated when people acknowledged my grieving and were patient with me.

Getting Out

I virtually lived in one room from October 18, 1996 to March 30, 1998. I had excursions out—I taught class and went to the store, but even then, my mind was in the room with Diana.

After she died, I felt strange being outside the room—not strange about being outside physically, but mentally. I had spent eighteen months thinking, "How do I keep her alive? How do I help her to recover? How do I make life better for her?" Suddenly, these thoughts had no relevance.

In the weeks after the funeral, Julie and my children knew I was struggling to regain my confidence in getting out. Julie dropped by and asked me to take a walk. It felt so strange to walk up High Street with nothing to do but walk and talk. Brendan asked me over to help him finish his basement, to eat dinner, to watch movies. Glen and Marisa asked for my help in building their deck. John invited me to Kentucky and to vacation with him in Cancun where it took me four days before I felt comfortable talking to strangers. Without these and similar invitations, I would be a basket case.

During the first few months after the funeral, several thoughts pestered me like begging children. Because I had been in a life-and-death struggle, I saw everything else as frivolous. It took me months to see recreation as rest and not a waste of precious time. Whenever I saw a couple or a family, I felt out of place. I wasn't yet single in my mind, and I clearly wasn't married—the vows were "Till death do us part." I was in no-man's land, feeling out of place with single people, married people, and families. All this took time.

I still teeter between "*we*" and "*I*". Is it really my house, my car, my family, my children—for there is no longer a "*we*"?

Was The Radiation and Chemotherapy Worth It?

My view of the benefits of radiation and chemotherapy has changed from the day after Diana's surgery to this writing. My opinion has become the opinion of the experienced—and, in many ways, the opinion held by doctors. I was most unhappy with the prognosis of one to three years, but the doctors were accurate—Diana split the difference and lived a little over 17 months. I was most unhappy with the prospect of her having to undergo radiation and chemotherapy, but these treatments gave us an additional year.

Was it worth it? Was the additional year worth the pain she went through? I've come to agree with Dr. Binder's view that any decision we make is the right decision—simply because there are no cures—and to choose to live longer with disabilities is equal to living shorter with abilities. In addition, no one knew or could predict Diana's condition after radiation. Most people thought she would have a period of weakness, nausea, perhaps vomiting, depression, and weight loss. But who would have thought she would have come close to death only to be blind and bedridden for a year?

If Diana had chosen only surgery, she probably would have died in the spring of 1997. She would not have seen our grandchildren. Then again, believing what I believe about souls, I think she would have met them in the spirit world—soul to soul.

We chose radiation because of a great number of choices over the years, choices that respected the achievements of traditional medicine while exploring the claims of alternative medicine. Our ties to traditional medicine were strong, Diana had seriously considered medical school, and our first son is a doctor. We had been ahead of traditional medicine in our approach to nutrition and vitamins. Only recently, for instance, have the minimum daily requirements been adjusted to reflect our thinking and practice. But we were also aware that alternative medicine was more preventative than curative, and that when you face an emergency you need emergency medicine. Traditional medicine is best for that.

Between vitamins and emergency medicine is a whole world of undeveloped traditional and alternative medicine, where traditional medicine is prone to the quick fix with little patient participation, and alternative medicine is prone to wishful thinking with too much patient participation. This middle ground is the new frontier where traditional and alternative medicine work together as partners, not competitors, and where funding for research is equitably distributed.

People often ask me if I would choose surgery, radiation, and chemotherapy if I had brain cancer. This is a good but hard question. While other forms of cancer are being treated successfully, brain cancer is not, at least as of this writing. As stated in the Informed Consent form, "Unfortunately, this type of cancer is almost never cured with surgery, radiation, or chemotherapy (drugs)."

Based on what Diana went through, if I got brain cancer I would choose surgery to give me a few months, but I would forego radiation and chemotherapy because they are too unproven for my tastes. I would fight to stay alive as long as I could to see even one more day with the people love.

Looking Back

Diana was an extraordinary person and an extraordinary patient. She was solicitous of everyone who took care of her, and she made her caregivers look good. She asked others about my health and about how I was dealing with the whole situation emotionally. She was concerned about the traffic on Route 66 that Brendan and I rode back and forth to work. And she remembered in detail the ongoing lives of those who came to visit her. As Carol put it, "She went through the whole thing in her head and just did it. She saved a lot of people a lot of agony. She was so bright that the picture was always large. She never had tunnel vision. Diana was so positive about things because she didn't want to upset people.

Diana also took care of herself during her illness. She declined to listen to a radio program on dying because it was upsetting. Again, in Carol's words, "Diana did everything she could to ensure her recovery. She accepted what she had to do and did it. She never had a crying fit. She never lost it, she never complained. She never said, 'Why me?' but said "I hope it's just a bad day because I couldn't deal with a setback just yet.' She knew she couldn't do anything about things. She accepted things for the way they were. She did everything she could to last as long as she did."

"I'm not ready to give up on this just now," Diana would say.

Guiding Ideas

Three guiding ideas made daily caring for Diana much easier.

Paying Attention This idea comes from Zen. Zen, of course, stresses letting go of the mind and bringing a relaxed, steady, one-pointed, direct perception of reality to bear on the activity at hand. I cannot count the number of times each day when I said to myself, "Let go, pay attention." If a thought, a memory, or a desire were getting in the way of my seeing clearly, I would let it go and bring my attention back to the task at hand. I remember doing this every time I washed Diana's face bringing my attention to focus on moving the washcloth across her forehead, her cheek, her nose, her eye, her chin, her upper lip, her ear, her neck. When I did this with full attention, Diana said she felt loved.

Research I observed, as a participant observer, the things I did for Diana. At times, I took written notes, but mostly, because of time constraints, I took mental notes. I reviewed these notes regularly—often at the end of the day but more often when I performed the same activity the following day. If something were not working, I tried to think of things to do to make it work. There were countless examples of this, such as when Diana said that her lower back was uncomfortable. I checked the sheets, the chucks and towels, the egg-crate mattress, and the bed. I noticed that the mattress was sliding down each time we raised the bed, so I placed a pillow between the footboard and the mattress. I also noticed that the egg-crate mattress was pressed flat under her hips and bottom. I inserted an extra strip of foam that had come with the mattress. This worked.

Refinement Jim Gray, founder of the National Writing Project, developed the project in 1974 and, over the years, modified it while keeping its basic principles. He called these modifications refinements. To me, refinements are small improvements made on a continuing basis. When Diana began feeding herself after going blind, she had trouble keeping the food on her plate. I bought large pasta bowls that gave her a rim against which to push the food onto her spoon. Julie also brought over a plastic guard that snapped on to the rim of the plate, and Diana used this until she mastered pushing the food against the rim.

These three ideas improved Diana's care, and made each day, in the best sense of the word, exciting.

Writing about Diana On January 21, 1997, I recorded the following in my journal:

> Diana asked me this morning if I were going to write about her situation. I don't know. Where would I start? It has been one of the most defining moments of my life.
>
> I could do a map but why would I want to write about this? It is so horrible. Yes, there are moments of joy and endearment, but there are also moments of sheer terror.

I wrote very little about Diana when she was alive—jotting down only a few things in my journal. It not only made me nauseous to write about her illness, I couldn't afford the time taken away from taking care of her.

After Diana died, I had no intention of writing about her. It wasn't until I got some distance and realized that she had led an extraordinary life in her last year, a life worth recording for all who knew her and members of the family who might come along later. I also realized we had been through a lot, and that our experiences might help others who find themselves in a similar situation.

The writing has forced me to open doors I might have kept closed for years. It has been an excellent way for me to grieve. It has helped me to think through and take a position on our choices and decisions I hope that this book has brought light into the lives of those who have read it.

I'll end with something Diana would often say to me as I left her to go downstairs, something that made me smile each time she said it, something that resonates with me even now, reminding me to live fully aware and in the present:

"Watch out for the cats on the stairs."

We both wanted our lives to go on after she died, to work through the past, and to live in the present. She has been so supportive in my doing just that, and I hope I have enabled her to do it as well.